Praise for *The Vibration of Grace*

"*The Vibration of Grace* is a rigorous blueprint for spiritual healing through the power of sound and soul. In this world, music is the meeting place and the resting place, and the place of transformation. Some practices allow you to go as deep as you think you can, while others gently invite you to get acquainted with who you are when nobody else is listening so you finally hear the beauty of your own true voice."

PEARL CLEAGE
Poet Laureate, City of Atlanta; author of
Some Things I Never Thought I'd Do

"gina Breedlove's voice and story are a vehicle for transformative change. Within the pages of *The Vibration of Grace*, gina takes you by the hand as she cracks open the most vulnerable pieces of herself and journeys into self-healing, freedom, and joy, using the powerful gifts of sound, self, and Grace. More than a 'how to,' this is a 'surrender to' the infinite possibilities of our own power to reclaim what we believed to be lost, and heal generational trauma in the process."

GINA TORRES
actor and producer

"The times we are living through demand that we have instructions and rituals that remind us that the wars being waged are not ours to win. gina Breedlove offers a manual for allowing our own grief to guide us home so that the instructions and rituals we receive are written by and belong to each of us. It would be easy to say that a gift as grand and generous as what gina Breedlove has called forth is breathtaking, but that would be too easy here. *The Vibration of Grace* is breath… and life-giving."

REV. ANGEL KYODO WILLIAMS
coauthor of *Radical Dharma*

T0049722

"gina Breedlove truly knows the beauty and power of sound and song. She offers moving stories of healing, as well as practical rituals—meditations, baths, journal prompts, and vocal practices—that enable readers to gently get in touch with their true selves and find spiritual recovery. Turn to this book for working with grief and anger, releasing fear, finding and giving forgiveness, and reconnecting with your soul. The advice here is shared to help address both the personal traumas as well as deep-seated societal harms that affect whole communities and, indeed, the planet."

TAMARA Y. JEFFRIES
senior editor, Yoga Journal

"What if you could reclaim your every breath? What if each breath you took from now on was a choir of ancestors reminding you how sacred each moment of your life is? It is impossible to overstate the generosity of this book. Thank you, gina, for making your many years of healing and teaching accessible in a form that can meet us right where we need it."

ALEXIS PAULINE GUMBS, PHD
author of *Undrowned*

"The healing and restorative power of sound frequency allows our bodies to release the tonic chemicals and endorphins needed for well-being, regeneration, and wholeness. If you are experiencing a healing journey, allow the wisdom, rituals, and practices in *The Vibration of Grace* to be your trusted guide."

MICHAEL BERNARD BECKWITH
founder and CEO of Agape International Spiritual Center,
author of *Life Visioning* and *Spiritual Liberation*

the
VIBRATION
of
GRACE

the
VIBRATION
of
GRACE

Sound Healing Rituals
for Liberation

gina Breedlove

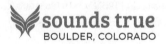
sounds true
BOULDER, COLORADO

Sounds True
Boulder, CO

Published 2023

Cover design by Huma Ahktar
Book design by Meredith Jarrett
Cover photo by Deadra M. Bryant

Printed in the United States of America

BK06751

Library of Congress Cataloging-in-Publication Data
Names: Breedlove, gina, author.
Title: The vibration of Grace : sound healing rituals for liberation /
   by gina Breedlove.
Description: Boulder, CO : Sounds True, 2023. |
   Includes bibliographical references.
Identifiers: LCCN 2023011361 (print) | LCCN 2023011362 (ebook) | ISBN
9781649631596 (trade paperback) | ISBN 9781649631602 (ebook)
Subjects: LCSH: Music therapy. | Rites and ceremonies. | Singing. |
   Healing.
Classification: LCC ML3920 .B615 2023 (print) | LCC ML3920 (ebook) |
   DDC 615.8/5154--dc23/eng/20230522
LC record available at https://lccn.loc.gov/2023011361
LC ebook record available at https://lccn.loc.gov/2023011362

10 9 8 7 6 5 4 3 2 1

For Valerie Jean Boyd, our most brilliant, beloved friend. Thank you, dear heart. You have left an indelible fragrance and a blazing trail of wonders to behold.

This Is How You Know That You Are God

All your traumas kneel and call you Saviour.

—KOLEKA PUTUMA, COLLECTIVE AMNESIA

Contents

Rituals

***Audio recordings of these practices are available at
soundstrue.com/vibration-of-grace-bonus**

Medicine Baths

Introduction

Grace and the Power of Sound: Your Body Is Your Sanctuary

D ear family, welcome to this journey. Let me tell you about the space you are entering. In this book you will receive detailed instruction and guidance for rituals and daily practices that will help you honor and release grief, fear, and anger from your body using the sound of your voice, your imagination, and the power of intention. You will learn how to work with the ancient ritual of soul retrieval to navigate trauma and past harm, gathering and liberating parts of yourself that may be caught in contorted positions. You will read testimonials from people I have been privileged to guide, who work with these rituals as an integral part of their well-being practice, and I will share with you my own story of healing and reclamation of my body, spirit, and mind from sexual trauma, abandonment, and anxiety. This book is a channeled work; most of the rituals shared here I have received from a being, a presence revealed to me as Grace. *The Vibration of Grace* is the healing energy inside these revolutionary practices that can teach you how to make your body a place of respite, where you may revel in feelings of ease, satisfaction, and freedom.

There is also wisdom here from my many years of service as a sound-healing practitioner. When sharing these rituals for well-being, I will sometimes say "we," which means the information is from me and Grace. We pray that this book will be of profound service to all who are seeking new pathways to personal agency and liberation from narratives that diminish and destroy what we seek to create. Let the space between us be open and blessed. May your ancestors and mine guide us through each ritual of grief-letting and reclamation, to a place of sovereignty and dominion over our lives.

This offering was channeled to remind you of the limitless, incalculable power you possess. To *channel* is to serve as a medium, a conduit for spirit. There are many opposing thoughts and opinions about channeling. I will not use our time together to debate or defend this practice. Grace tells me that we all have the capacity to receive messages from spirit. I trust Grace, and I trust your intuition. If you are drawn to this book, there is medicine here for you. You do not need to have experience with channeling to engage with these rituals, and the practices you will find here are not offered to create the experience of channeling. We invite you to focus on deepening your own healing practice. The only things you will need to work with this book are curiosity, willingness, and time.

The Vibration of Grace invites you to expand your understanding of the medicine that exists inside you and your capacity to govern your own healing. We begin by introducing rituals to identify your soul tones, the sound of you, your personal resonance and vibration. We then guide you through the power of affirmations to shape, shift, and anchor your desires for your life. These are foundational learnings that will support you as you practice rituals to release the grief that can get caught in the body.

Grief is an emotional, physical, and spiritual response to loss. Grieving is a powerful and potentially cathartic process that so many of us are taught to stifle, swallow, and ignore. Grief is energy that wants to be let. It needs expression and a pathway out of the body so that it does not ossify and become something hard and brittle that takes up residence in our psyche, internal organs, and blood. We are surrounded by glorious examples of service, solutions, beauty, and care, created from a place of grieving. This book will guide you into the sanctuary that is your body to where you may be storing grief and teach you how to release grief by using the sound of your voice and the power of your mind-body wisdom.

We are currently working on rituals to serve people who are deaf, hard of hearing, nonspeaking, or may have speech disabilities. In this book, many of the rituals require being able to make and hear sound. Please feel welcome to adapt these rituals to your own accessibility needs as you are guided by your spirit.

The rituals we offer here are structured similarly in each chapter to help set a strong container for your work. You will find instructions that guide you with *Tools*, *Preparation*, *Ritual*, and *Closing*. Within this template, there may be elements that are unique; adjustments can be made particular to your accessibility needs. There is a sound-healing ritual for group work, a pulling practice to dispel another person's energy from your body, a ritual to replenish the energy in your vital organs, meditation, breathwork, affirmations, practices that teach the art of true apology, and recipes for medicinal baths (please check to make sure all ingredients for the baths will not conflict with any medicines you may be taking).

During each ritual, please do not use recorded music unless we invite you to do so. Lyrics and instrumental compositions can be distracting and pull focus. We place *you and your accessibility needs* at the center of each solo ritual. When doing circle work, we take turns centering each individual present and learn how our personal needs may coexist to support each other. Please follow our guidance as closely as you can to receive the intended benefits.

We close *The Vibration of Grace* with a glossary to support deeper understanding, as well as "Recommended Resources," where you will find a list of practitioners and organizations involved in all manner of healing and a reading list of beautiful, nourishing books that help us love ourselves and each other in all the ways.

Audio Guide of Ritual Instruction

Here is the link to an audio guide of my voice supporting you through some of the rituals: soundstrue.com/vibration-of-grace-bonus.

Before engaging with the audio guide to the rituals, please read or listen through the chapter you're working with so you will have all the tools needed and complete the required preparation. The audio guide to the rituals allows us to take our time, breathe together, and engage fully, bringing all of ourselves to the moment.

The Power of Sound

The medicine of Grace is sound. Sound has an immediate point of entry to the mind, body, and spirit. Sound creates vibration, an energy that shapes and moves everything. Grace tells me that sound has been sourced as a healing modality since humans appeared on the earth. The Vedas, ancient Hindu scriptures, contain thousands of mantras that create vibrational frequencies when chanted that impact the neurons in the body. All over the world are resonating structures that amplify the power of sound, such as ancient Mayan temples, Egyptian pyramids, Stonehenge (which hums when the wind blows just so), and caves in Utah, New Mexico, and Peru, to name a few. The medicine of sound is shared in many ways, including using drums, didgeridoo, bells, chanting, prayers, crystal bowls, and when singing along to your favorite song, which may also cause you to dance and feel better. The sounds of the natural world can help us to remember beauty: rushing rivers, quiet streams, oceans, rain, birds singing, children laughing, and so many more.

The healing effects of sound on the body can be explained in scientific terminology too. A cranial nerve called the vagus nerve, the longest nerve in the body, impacts almost every major organ. It is connected to your vocal cords, the muscles at the back of your throat, and passes through your inner ear. The vagus nerve is the main nerve of the parasympathetic nervous system and connected to your larynx (voice box), so that whenever you sing, hum, and speak, the nerve is activated. Internally created sound has a direct effect on our internal systems. There are myriad documented studies by neurologists and scientists on the healing effects sound and frequency have on the human body, such as using acoustics to manipulate cells or using an apparatus that translates brain activity into sound to detect seizures, listening to the blood to monitor blood pressure, using sound waves to disrupt the growth of cancerous cells, and humming to calm the parasympathetic nervous system.[1]

Grace has shared with me that the millions of pores that cover our body are more than exit points for oil and sweat; pores are also openings that receive sound. Those of us who have been working with sound as a healing modality through the guidance of spirit already know what is being reconfirmed and remembered by science: sound and vibration are indeed potent and powerful healing modalities.

Your Voice

The sound of your voice and the energy of your presence are as personal as your fingerprint and carry a vibrational frequency that uniquely belongs to you. The shape of your mouth, the placement and size of your vocal cords, tongue, larynx, the capacity of your lungs, how many languages you use: there are many things that make your voice yours. The voice also carries inherent awareness and evidence of lineage. Many of us do not know our ancestors, but as with blood, there is power inside of your sound and a connection to those in your lineage who have come before you.

Our cells respond to sound. The sound of your voice and the power of vibration married with intention can produce an immediate effect on your being. Even if you don't enjoy or have access to the sound of your voice, you can learn how to source the medicinal effect of toning, tapping, humming, chanting, and affirming. You do not need to think of yourself as a singer to practice sound healing.

---

1   Roberto M. Soriano, Ryan Winters, and Vikas Gupta, "Anatomy, Head and Neck: Larynx Nerves," National Center for Biotechnology Information, September 18, 2022, ncbi.nlm.nih.gov/books/NBK557742/; Nathan Collins, "Stanford researchers listen for silent seizures with 'brain stethoscope' that turns brain waves into sound," Stanford News, March, 20, 2018, news.stanford.edu/2018/03/20/brain-stethoscope-listens-silent-seizures/; Elana Gordon, "The sounds of blood pressure: What are we listening for?" February 8, 2016, "WHYY" on PBS/NPR, whyy.org/articles/the-sounds-of-blood-pressure-what-are-they-listening-for/.

About Grace and Me

I am about to share a personal story that includes abandonment. Please take care of yourself and feel welcome to come back to this section at another time.

The first time I heard Grace speak I was six years old, standing on the front steps of our apartment building in Crown Heights, Brooklyn, in 1971. I was watching my mother leave, driving away in a car I had never seen before with a man I had never met. I watched the car go for a long time, waiting for my mother to return. I knew she wasn't coming back, and I waited anyway. My four siblings and my father were upstairs in our apartment. It seemed to me they were unaware of what had just happened.

My father was sitting in his usual spot on the couch, staring into space, a pile of empty beer cans growing around his feet. My sisters and brothers, the older two and the younger two, were watching television in the room with my father, finding solace in *The Partridge Family*, a show about a family of traveling musicians making their way around the world on a brightly colored tour bus with a happy ending at the close of each episode.

Anchored to the doorstep, I could not make myself return to the apartment. Our mother had just moved out and I had helped her downstairs with her luggage. Holding vigil on the front steps with feelings that were too big for my six-year-old body, I heard Grace say: *Sing, gina. Sing and you will feel better. Sing right now.* I began to sing the chorus of the song "La La Means I Love You" by the Delfonics softly to myself, soothing my heart with the sweet, simple beauty of the melody and the promise inside the words. The sound of my voice broke the spell of feeling stuck. I sang myself off the stoop, up the stairs to the second floor, and into our house of immense grief. I found my way to the top bunk bed and sang and cried until I fell asleep.

Throughout my life, Grace has been a constant presence, a calm and steady knowing at the center of my being. Although the name Grace is associated with feminine pronouns, I have been guided to refer to Grace as "They" and "We." During my sound-healing sessions, Grace will address community as "family." When Grace speaks, their voice is like an inner echo moving through my spirit, distinguishable by the absolute clarity of the instruction for rituals and concepts that I personally have no reference for. With Grace's guidance, I have returned to that Brooklyn doorstep often to rescue my six-year-old self and practiced rituals of soul retrieval and trance work, discovering this language as my work deepened.

After years of practicing sound healing on my own body, Grace told me that I could also help others. I began to offer private sound-healing sessions in 2008. The testimonies shared here are from people I've worked with over the years, guiding them back to themselves using all the rituals in this book. With their permission and preferred pronouns, we share their stories to dispel narratives of isolation and to show what is possible.

When requests for private sessions began to exceed space on my calendar, I asked Grace how this work could be made available for more people. Thus, this book was born.

Grace and Ownership of Self

Grace tells me that our body is our primary home. She asks us to ask ourselves, *Do I own my mind?* There is a constant campaign for our consciousness, where we place our attention, who and what we believe, what we dream about. It seems that most conversations we have with each other are peppered with what is *trending*. In this work, the path to liberation begins with focusing on ourselves, turning toward the questions: *Do I own my mind? Do I think the thoughts I wish to think? Do I trust the sound of my own voice? Do I feel at home in my body? The Vibration of Grace* can teach you how to embrace your own body wisdom, as your unfettered mind remembers who you are and what you desire for your life.

We are living in a time of great opportunity and danger. There exists an energy of undoing that can steal our will and weaken our capacity to imagine and create a world that truly cares for everyone.

And Grace tells me that love will always prevail. I gratefully align my energy and voice with the many, many humans around the planet working for liberation, justice, and freedom for all beings. I have personally tended to some of these folks, helping them to stay well inside of their incredible output of energy toward a healing world. I have sat in rooms with organizers, healers, and community members, where the fight for reproductive justice, transgender and LGBTQIA rights, the Movement 4 Black Lives (M4BL), language justice, land justice, and climate justice are living, breathing acts of persistence. And I have been privileged to teach and learn from the brilliance of younger people who are trying to make the world a better place for all beings. We have much repair work to do, within ourselves and our interconnected communities, and there is ample reason to feel hopeful. We can heal as we fight to dismantle horrific, destructive systems and respond to the needs of our collective present moment without constantly feeling overwhelmed and exhausted.

A sound healing practice is one way to caretake your body as we move beside each other on this long journey to true freedom. Sound is also a healing modality that pairs beautifully with other well-being practices and guided medicine journeys designed for healing: somatic therapy, Reiki, acupuncture, ayahuasca, psilocybin therapy, and EMDR, to name just a few.

Daily Practice

The essential requirement for these rituals to be most effective is practice. *The Vibration of Grace* is about caring for yourself from your marrow to your skin, and to fully embrace these rituals will mean that you have to release old patterns and behaviors, which requires focus and time. Daily practice should be tailored to suit your life: a half hour of ritual each morning to begin your day, an evening practice before you close your eyes to rest at night. There are also rituals here that you can engage throughout your day, like noticing beauty and humming, or pausing to take five deep breaths before that next call. Practice is key to our salvation. Practice is how we heal.

As you move beyond this introduction, you are invited to read this book in a linear way; please know that on the opening page of parts 1, 2, 3, and 4, I've included snippets of lyrics from songs I've written. You can also fast-forward to a chapter that speaks to you, or allow yourself to be divinely guided by holding the book in your hands, closing or softening your eyes, breathing deeply for a few minutes, and asking out loud, "What do I need to know today?" Then open to a page—a seemingly random choice that invariably will be just the thing you need to see, read, know, and share.

Dear family, we are grateful to meet you here. May you be covered in love.

part one

FOUNDATION
—— *for your* ——
SOUND PRACTICE

we want to give you something, to have to hold
we wish to give you something, this path to the soul
the light in your eyes, your breath and your skin
and all the power that lies within . . .

1

Sound and Your Soul Tones:
The Key of You

Dear family, we begin with rituals for remembering and working with your soul tones, the sounds that emanate from the living, breathing presence that is you. Your soul tones come from marrow-deep medicine and wisdom housed within your cells, ancestral and spiritual legacies, and an inheritance of limitlessness. They are sounds that you embody, often described as vibrational presence, the energy you bring into a room. A daily practice of humming or singing your soul tones to yourself can help you feel an immediate sense of calm and groundedness. We are surrounded by a cacophony of sounds that can feel like noise, and we forget or don't know how to experience our own resonance. Your soul tones are sounds you can reach for when you need to gather yourself. They can support you as you move through the grief-letting rituals in this book, providing opportunity to pause and breathe.

We rediscover our soul tones by leaning into the sounds we are most drawn to. For our shared practice, we will work with the eight musical notes of the C-major scale and nine solfeggio frequencies. Solfeggio frequencies are specific tones that carry sound medicine for healing the mind, spirit, and body.

Universally, we share sound, so your soul tones can be the same note or frequency as someone else's. What makes your soul tones particular to you is how the sound moves within your body, spirit, and mind. Like the limbs and leaves of a tree joined at the root, our lives are both interconnected and individual, anchored in the shared language of love and consciousness that becomes part of our soul tones. This collective wisdom stays with us throughout our lives, beneath our stories, experiences, and learnings, to be remembered when we are ready. Sometimes on the edge of daybreak, we will wake to hear our soul tones reminding us of the truth of our being, our place in the interwoven layering of everything.

The "everything" is love. It keeps the earth orbiting the sun and the moon pulling on the tides. Love is why all the horror that has happened in this realm has not extinguished hope. It is the reason we live, why we are here. Love is a verb, being, force, presence—love is everything. And love has a sound that imbues our soul tones. This is something we all have in common—all of us, not some of us—and it creates the possibility for us to recognize each other's humanity, even in terrible conditions.

We understand that for many, love is a difficult being. Our intention is not to diminish or deny anyone's personal journey, but to provide tools, a set of rituals, that can support our combined efforts to heal and co-create a world that shelters and cares for all. This practice of loving each other is linked to the practice of loving ourselves. Living into our soul tones enhances all of our practices because it can ground us in self-awareness, which helps us to remember our power. Soul tones are also how we recognize each other when we meet again.

Soul Tones and Transmigration

I know from Grace that all beings travel together across lifetimes, shaping each other, choosing to meet again and again in new incarnations, to evolve in and as love, to become fluent in the language of light. When two souls are drawn to each other, they are keeping an appointment to continue a learning process, honoring invisible agreements. When there is an immediate feeling of familiarity, our soul tones are aligning in harmonious ways; however, the harmonious feeling of soul tones aligned does not dictate what the relationship and learnings will be. These reunions can be glorious, painful, thrilling, difficult, and sometimes all these things in one journey. Expansion happens when the relationship inspires us to grow. Sometimes grief is the catalyst for change, and other times learning to receive joy is the catalyst. Often, these relationships will keep us living into our growing edge, giving us opportunities to deepen and learn more about love.

You may already be leaning into your soul tones daily, listening to the music that moves your spirit. When you listen to the songs you love, notice similarities in melody and the overall vibe. Notice the notes in the song that you wait for each time, that make you dance, cry, feel. The whole song may give you life and help you to come home to yourself, as music is amazing medicine. Working with your soul tones is a practice you can lean into for immediate care you may need at any given moment. It is one antidote for the stress that can rise when you're faced with an unexpected challenge.

——————— Ritual ———————
FOR FINDING YOUR SOUL TONES

The intention with this practice is to identify the sound or sounds that create an immediate sense of calm within your body because they match the sounds your presence emits, your soul tones. For our beginning practice, you will be working with the eight musical notes of the C-major scale and nine solfeggio frequencies. There are 48 major and minor scales, with the pentatonic (five-note) scale—the most commonly used scale in music throughout the world. We begin with the C-major scale because I have found it to be the simplest point of entry when teaching this ritual. In the audiobook of *The Vibration of Grace* and the audio guide to each ritual, we will share the C-major scale and the solfeggio frequencies with this practice. Otherwise, you will need to source the C-major scale via the internet or use a musical instrument to play the scale. To begin, you will choose one note and one solfeggio frequency to work with. You can do the following rituals on the same day and work with them simultaneously, or you can complete one and then the other.

Tools

- internet access on a phone, computer, tablet, etc.

- a journal

Preparation

The first part of this ritual usually takes an hour. In the days to follow, you will be practicing the ritual throughout the whole day. Decide what date you will begin this practice and mark *seven* days forward on your calendar for a total of *eight* days. Open your journal and copy the C-major scale and solfège written in bold print below. You may be familiar with solfège, a system of learning musical scales (and the C-major scale) from the song "Do-Re-Mi" in the movie *The Sound of Music*. Solfège (DO, RE, MI, FA, SOL, LA, TI, DO) is above the accompanying notes (C, D, E, F, G, A, B, C) below:

DO	RE	MI	FA	SOL	LA	TI	DO
C	D	E	F	G	A	B	C

Open a computer, phone, or other device you use to access the internet and locate an audio example of a simple C-major scale using solfège. I like this offering you can find on YouTube.com from Corix Music titled "Do Re Mi Ear Training Exercise/Technique (C Major)"; it's a continuous practice of ascending and descending the scale. Listen to the C-major scale on repeat until you can hum or sing along.

Ritual

Sitting comfortably with your back supported or standing with your knees slightly bent and legs hip-width apart, soften or close your eyes and bring your awareness to your breath. If you are standing and it feels good to you, allow your body to sway gently from side to side. Inhale deeply through your nose and exhale audibly through your mouth, slowly, for *five* complete breaths. After the *fifth* exhale, continue with the breathing practice as you guide your awareness to the back of your skull, the back of your neck, then the shoulders, and down your spine, vertebrae by vertebrae, until you reach your sacrum (the base of your spine), and pause here for *two* complete breaths. Inhaling and exhaling, guide your awareness to your perineum, the space between your anus and genitals, and then travel up the front of your body, past your navel, stomach, and the center of your chest, to the base of your throat. Keep your thoughts there while you take *five* more complete breaths, inhaling deeply through your nose and exhaling through your mouth.

Feel Each Note: When you're ready, begin to sing solfège, following the C-major scale, repeating each note slowly *five* times. You can sing softly so that only you can hear, or be loud about it—it is your choice. Practice focusing on the sound, and notice if and how your body responds. Record this information in your journal, and then move on to the next note. If you have trouble singing or humming a note, stay with your breath practice while you listen deeply to each note on your device. If you are singing, your practice will look like this:

> Inhale deeply, exhale DOOOOOOOOO to the end of your breath; do this *five* times, then journal.
>
> Inhale deeply, exhale REEEEEEEEEE to the end of your breath; do this *five* times, then journal.
>
> Inhale deeply, exhale MIIIIIIIIIIIIIIIII to the end of your breath; do this *five* times, then journal.
>
> Inhale deeply, exhale FAAAAAAAAA to the end of your breath; do this *five* times, then journal.
>
> Inhale deeply, exhale SOOOOOOOOO to the end of your breath; do this *five* times, then journal.
>
> Inhale deeply, exhale LAAAAAAAAA to the end of your breath; do this *five* times, then journal.
>
> Inhale deeply, exhale TIIIIIIIIIIIIIIIIII to the end of your breath; do this *five* times, then journal.
>
> Inhale deeply, exhale DOOOOOOOOO to the end of your breath; do this *five* times, then journal.

Choose Your High-Vibration Word: When you have worked with all eight notes of the major scale, choose the one your body has the most favorable response to and marry this note with a word whose meaning has a high vibrational energy, like the words *joy, peace*, or *grace*. Work with the note and the word you have chosen throughout each day for one week. You can also try different words, but stay with the same note. For example, if you find that singing FA (F) is the note that slows down your breath and relaxes your shoulders, choose a word (mine would be *grace*) and sing that word to the tone of FA (F) to yourself as you move through your day. I work with this practice when I wake, while sitting with my morning coffee, walking, driving, and when I pause to look up and appreciate the sky. Your word song may be sung in long notes or in tandem with the rhythm of your beating heart—you choose.

Closing

When you wake on the *ninth* day, make time that morning to sit with your journal and reflect on your eight days of practice. Write down your thoughts, discoveries, what you noticed, and answer these questions:

- Which note resonated most in your being?
- Which word did you work with?
- Why?
- How did this ritual serve you?

After answering these questions, honor yourself for completing this eight-day practice. Write your own words of praise for yourself in your journal or use mine, and speak them aloud so your spirit may receive them:

"I am grateful for the beautiful sound inside of my soul and the wisdom that my body holds. I am a powerful being."

Return to your journaling and ask yourself if you have any questions about the practice you've completed. Write them down. You may discover the answers in this book as you keep reading.

Once you have mastered the C-major scale practice, I encourage you to explore the major pentatonic scale—my personal favorite, five sounds of gorgeous possibility.

You can engage this practice as often as you wish. I keep my soul tones cycling through my being daily, humming to myself, thinking, and speaking a good word to my spirit, which fortifies my being and helps me to stay embodied.

—————————— Ritual ——————————

FOR SOLFEGGIO FREQUENCIES AS SOUL TONES

There are many theories about the origin of the solfeggio frequencies. Grace tells me that these sounds and all notes are part of the fabric of the everything, which is always singing. Some sounds are pitched beyond our capacity to hear with our ears, though we feel them in our being. Musical notes and frequencies are channeled from the multiverse for collective grace. And you do not have to know the origin story of these sounds to receive the benefits of this holy offering.

For sourcing soul tones, I prefer to work with the pure sound of each frequency. In our audiobook and the accompanying audio guide to the rituals, pure tones for each solfeggio frequency are offered. If not through one of these, you will need to access the internet to source these sounds.

Tools

- internet access on a computer, phone, tablet, etc.
- a journal
- a recording device
- a timer

Preparation

Open your journal and write down your answers to these questions:

- How are you feeling?
- Do you have any experience working with solfeggio frequencies?

You will be using your journal during this ritual, so have it close by before you begin your meditation. The beginning of this practice will generally require about sixty minutes to complete. Once you choose the solfeggio frequency your body responds to, you will work with this sound throughout your day for *five* days. As I've already mentioned, if you do not have access to our audio offerings, you will need to use the internet to locate videos that offer a pure tone for each solfeggio frequency. For example, to search online for the first frequency, you would enter the search term "174 Hz pure tone" to find an audio recording. When you're done with one frequency, move on to the next frequency listed. During the ritual, you will be listening to each tone for *two* minutes.

Ritual

Sitting comfortably with your back supported or standing with your knees slightly bent and legs hip-width apart, soften or close your eyes and bring your full awareness to your breath. Inhale deeply, and as slowly as you are able, exhale audibly. Repeat this breath practice for *five* full breaths. Take a mental journey from the soles of your feet to your knees, thighs, perineum, navel, stomach, chest, base of the throat, forehead, to the top of your skull—all the while staying with your breath practice. Then from the top of your skull, breathe as you guide your awareness down your back body, past your beating heart on the left side, your liver on the right, your kidneys anchoring your spine, your sacrum, the backs of your thighs, your calves, and once again to the soles of your feet. Breathe.

Open your journal and prepare to write your experience of listening and feeling each pure tone. Write down this list of the frequencies in your journal:

174 Hz	417 Hz	741 Hz
285 Hz	528 Hz	852 Hz
396 Hz	639 Hz	963 Hz

If you are working with a computer, locate each pure tone online. Please try not to read or listen to descriptions of what the sound is for; instead, lean into your body's response and have your own experience of the solfeggio frequencies. We will return to each frequency at the end of the ritual to learn what those who have been working with the frequencies for many years have found. It is important to allow your own body wisdom to respond to this offering without a preconceived knowing.

Let us begin: Set your timer for *two* minutes, and listen to the first tone with your eyes closed or with your eyes softened and your gaze unfocused. When the timer chimes, stop the sound and pause to consider your body's response. Breathe deeply, inhaling through your nose and exhaling through your mouth. Open your journal and write your reflections. Then listen to the next tone using the same guidelines, until you have listened and written about all *nine* frequencies.

After you complete your first pass of listening and writing, close your journal. Then listen again to each solfeggio frequency for *two* minutes (using your timer). During each listen, inhale deeply and exhale through your mouth. Feel the effect of the tone on your body and spirit. Try not to think about it; instead, stay with your breath practice and listen with as little focused thought as possible. If your mind tries to lead you elsewhere, pause the sound and turn your attention to breathing. When you are ready, return to the sound and listen. Once you have completed your listening, choose the tone that resonates most in your being. This is the sound that is aligning with your soul tones. If you have trouble choosing, open your journal and read what you have written for each tone; choose the tone that had the most impact.

Now that you've chosen, you will listen to this frequency daily for *five* days. Record the sound using a cell phone or another recording device, so that you can easily access it throughout your day. You can even listen while you sleep if you wish. Some online sources, including those I list in "Recommended Resources" near the back of this book, provide eight hours of listening for each frequency. I don't like to sleep with a computer near my head, so when I listen to a solfeggio tone while sleeping, I place the computer far from my pillow and put the volume on low. If you listen while sleeping, write about the experience in your journal the next morning.

If you're still unsure about which tone to choose, review this list that shares some of the meaning and healing intention behind each of the frequencies. Does one align with your current needs? If yes, that is the tone you will use for your ritual.

174 Hz - pain reduction and stress release
285 Hz - cellular repair
396 Hz - letting go of fear
417 Hz - clearing energetic blockages
528 Hz - heart opening and transformation
639 Hz - interconnection and community repair
741 Hz - activating intuition and clarity
852 Hz - consciousness and spirituality
963 Hz - oneness and enlightenment

Closing

On the *sixth* morning, notice how you are feeling. Open your journal and reread the entry you made before you began this practice. Write your answers to these questions:

- What feels different after five days of listening to the solfeggio tone?

- Was this ritual of service to you?

- How so?

Write down anything else you wish to record and remember. Then give yourself praise for completing this practice, and write this down. Create your own affirmation to honor your work, or use this one:

I am proud of myself for completing this ritual and deepening my connection to the powerful being that I AM.

Now that you have completed the two ritual practices and have worked with two sounds you have identified as soul tones, you can lean into these sounds at will. Continue to sing your word to yourself, using a note from the C-major scale, and listen to your solfeggio tone. If you wish, repeat the rituals and experiment with new notes and a different tone. Bring these sounds into your day-to-day by sounding your word softly to yourself, whether before a potentially difficult conversation or to extend a moment of ease. Source these sounds when you wish to change your mind about something. Sing your word to yourself when you feel afraid or unclear. Live into the sound of your own voice holding your life.

We are ready now to move into our grief-letting rituals. Your soul tones will support you in these practices, holding you as you hold them.

2

Sound and Affirmation: Your Language for Healing

Dear family, I'm about to talk about violence, addiction, and self-harm. Please take care of yourself. If you need to, you are welcome to go directly to the affirmations located at the end of this chapter.

I became aware of suicidal ideation around age eleven. It was a common thought among the people I knew in my circle of school and neighborhood friends. There was so much violence and addiction around us all the time, it seemed to us that none of us were going to live long anyway. Many of my friends had older siblings who were addicted to heroin, and years later, crack rolled through like a brush fire decimating communities.

Our saving grace was music, the affirmative sounds of Black music in the 1970s: "Songs in the Key of Life," an album by Stevie Wonder, was released the month we started sixth grade. This record was amazing and kept us dancing and singing in the school yard. The magic of every song Earth, Wind & Fire sang lifted our spirits to the clouds above and beyond. We listened to the Isley Brothers when we wanted to feel grown, giggling and dreaming about a first kiss and romantic love. And then there were songs that became anthems, calling us to solidarity and awareness, as we sang the chorus with fists pumping the air, feeling in those moments that anything and everything was possible. "Wake up Everybody," sung by Teddy Pendergrass and Harold Melvin & the Blue Notes, is a song about community healing and accountability, and it was the jam. The popular songs we listened to in my Brooklyn had a common energetic: love of self, love of family, and love of community. The lyrics to almost every song you heard were full of positive imagery and kept us believing in the possibility of a new day. The music and lyrics from my childhood introduced me to the power of affirmations.

During this time of navigating daily grief and encroaching puberty, Grace would tell me stories of a future full of love and joy for me and my community. I tried to share some of Grace's wisdom and sight with my siblings and friends, but they all told me I was ("crazy",) that I was hearing voices and that Grace was not real. Their doubt and ridicule caused a shift in my relationship with Grace. I felt isolated, and I was too young to understand that my siblings and friends were navigating their own feelings of grief and fear. I wondered if my five-year-old self had imagined the quiet, still voice that had been speaking to me since the day my mother left and if I really was losing my mind. Everyone treated me differently after I told them about Grace, as though maybe I thought I had some special talent and was above them in some way. This hurt my heart, and it was the first time that Grace's presence brought me sadness and confusion. I began to turn away from Grace's guidance. and after a while, the voice went quiet. I'd tried to share Grace's affirmation of what was possible for our lives, but I was met with resistance, because Grace was showing me a future that conflicted with our present reality, a future that my friends and family could not see, from a being that my friends and family could not see.

A week before my thirteenth birthday and a month after my father's passing, my aunt brought me to see a Broadway show, a choreo-poem by Ntozake Shange called "for colored girls who have considered suicide / when the rainbow is enuf." It opened my mind and loosed my spirit. Seven luminous Black women together onstage, telling stories, laughing, dancing, crying, raging, talking about things I mostly did not understand, but I felt the power of their presence and words at the center of my being. I was particularly moved by the Lady in Blue, played by the astonishing Laurie Carlos. I could see myself reflected in this light-skinned Black woman who could sing. I wanted to be like her when I grew up. She gifted me with a new focus for my existence, nourished by witnessing what was possible for a Black girl from Brooklyn, or anywhere. I left the theater and promptly bought the book, the record, everything I could find with Ntozake Shange's name attached, for she was the creator of this work and the bringer of new light to my world. I was changed, again and again.

"i found god in myself and i loved her fiercely" became my mantra at thirteen; inspired by a line from a poem in *For colored girls who have considered suicide when the rainbow is enuf.* I felt the medicinal power in this statement: I felt emboldened and capable and real. I sang it, chanted it, wrote it in all my school notebooks. This affirmation floated me through my teenage years. This language from Ntozake Shange gave me a new sense of myself. And though we were still estranged, I felt the presence of Grace in this new knowing. I had been using humming to calm myself for years; with this affirmation, I discovered that I could also use words to own my body and the space I occupied. Poems and statements that began with "I AM" felt so powerful in my mouth and in my spirit. I had new armor that could protect me against any kind of trespass. I felt less afraid.

Grace returned to my consciousness when I was fifteen. I was on an F train heading toward Manhattan, on my way to the High School for the Performing Arts for my tenth-grade drama class. I was thinking about my academic classes when suddenly my heart began to race, my body began to sweat, and I felt dizzy, like I was going to pass out. I got off the train and found a seat and began to try to calm myself by humming and toning, the way Grace taught me. I was terrified that I might be losing my mind. My thoughts felt disjointed, crowding my reason. I had no language for anxiety attacks. Nothing like this had ever happened to me. I was deciding to go home when for the first time in about four years I heard Grace's voice, clearly inviting me to listen and get back on the train. All the way to 46th Street, I repeated the two sentences Grace spoke in my spirit, echoing the words aloud so that only I could hear:

I am strong, I am capable, I belong here.
I am alive, I am loved, I belong here.

When I got off the train to go to school, I had a clear knowing that if I had returned home, I would not have had the courage to go back. Grace guided me to expand my affirmation practice on that train, and I continue to practice to this day—shifting, releasing, and reprogramming core beliefs forged by sadness, by speaking affirmative language.

Power in the Word

Imagine for a moment that your breath is sacred and every word that you think and speak is imbued with this energy. Imagine that the meaning behind the word that has been thought and spoken is activated by your breath and becomes an energetic being that follows your focus and goes where you send it.

I heard our beloved poet, teacher, and renaissance woman Maya Angelou say that words are things and that one day we would be able to measure the power of words. My father, whose mother had said this to him, would also say this to me and my siblings when we were growing up. There is an intrinsic knowing about the mental and oracular power to create, transform, release, harm, bless, and welcome with words. I have seen how the energetic weight of unexpressed needs can harm the body, how a "no" not honored can weaken the spirit, while a "yes" given freely feels like seabirds in flight.

Breathe deeply now, please, inhaling through your nose and exhaling through your mouth. Take your time. Breathe and consider: What if this is true? What if breath, words, and intention have power? What would this mean to you and the words you choose? If we could see with our eyes the way words land on our skin, seeping through the pores, how the energy of what has been thought or said finds its way to the blood flow and internal organs, how would we speak to ourselves?

How Narratives Become

I grew up hearing that I was too much. Too emotional, too loud, too big, too chatty, too everything. These narratives became fused with my identity, and many of my choices and responses came from this place of thinking I was a burden. Affirmations helped me to heal and change these narratives. The truth has a sound and resonance our body responds to when we hear it spoken, even if our mind, armed with whatever narrative is waiting to co-opt the moment, will step in and take over to lead us away from what we know. Affirmations help us to change our minds, hone our listening skills, and dispatch the narratives that exist only to cause us harm.

Sometimes we need other kinds of support on our journey to heal our narratives. There are unadulterated medicines from the earth that can support those who need to delve deeper into their psyches to release an untruth. My path is not connected to teaching about these medicines, and I am not allowed to speak in detail of these beings that exist to heal humanity. I have had two journeys with the being Ayahuasca. They were incredibly beautiful experiences for me. If you are called, if you are guided to any plant-based medicine, find those who have been studying for many years to guide you. Make sure to research and know the lineage, the root, and the connection your teacher/guide has to the medicine that calls you. Ask your ancestors for guidance, consult with trusted community, and believe your intuition—the answers will come.

Affirmation Rituals

Leaning into the sound of my 13-year-old voice, hearing myself proclaim that God lived inside of me and I was worthy of fierce love, helped me to keep living. And midway through my 57th year, I still practice affirmations, sometimes daily. I give to myself what I give to others, the sound of my voice cheering me on, forever teaching me about love.

Tools

- a calendar
- a journal

Preparation

We are bombarded with promotions and promises for wellness, built around impossible timing: "In just seven days you can achieve . . ." or "Do this for 21 days and be healed of . . ."—fill in the blanks. I think we know by now that the quick fix is not a thing; it is not real.

As for affirmations, it can be helpful to create a set time to practice, to feel your way into how the affirmation you have chosen is working for you. For the purpose of a shared agreement, our timeline for this initial practice will be *fifteen* days. Open your calendar and choose a day to begin your affirmation practice, and count fifteen days forward. You will be practicing when you wake and before you go to sleep. You are welcome to use your affirmations throughout the day, while the commitment is to engage every morning and at bedtime.

When working with the affirmations, you will notice that we place emphasis on the words "I AM." We know that there is great power in a declarative statement. "I AM" also comes from Christian and Judaic holy books, detailing how God named and described itself.

Ritual

Begin and close each day listening to the sound of your voice, and feel the vibration of your beating heart. When you wake and open your eyes, guide your first thoughts to conscious breathing. Take *five* deep breaths, inhaling slowly through your nose and audibly exhaling through your mouth. Listen to your unhurried, untroubled breathing. Then say your affirmation to yourself out loud, as you rise from your rest and begin to prepare for your day. Do this practice before you reach for your phone, computer, daily planner, etc. Take at least *fifteen* minutes. Listen to your voice as you recite the words you have chosen for your morning practice; remember that you are to speak to yourself the way you speak to someone or some being that you love. You may also invite a beloved to record the affirmations you choose and lean into the sound of their voice each day.

When you are ready to go to sleep at night, turn off all devices at least a half hour before you plan to sleep. Bring your awareness to conscious breathing, inhaling through your nose and audibly exhaling through your mouth. Begin your affirmation as you prepare for bed. If possible, let the sound of your voice or the voice you have chosen to affirm you be the sound that carries you to sleep.

Here is a list of affirmations we believe will be of service to you. We have shared some that feel universal and some that may be specific to your vocation and present-moment happenings. It is possible that you may be drawn to an affirmation even if it does not feel specific to your life. Please be guided by your spirit. To begin, please choose *two* affirmations. After you become practiced here, you may work with more than one.

Universal Affirmations

- *I love myself and I will do all that I can to be more loving to myself.*

- *I always know which way to go; I trust my body's wisdom.*

- *I Am not ashamed of the life I chose; I revel in being myself.*

- *I Am worthy of being seen and loved for who I Am.*

- *I forgive everyone; everyone forgives me. I let go of grief, and I set myself free.*

- *My heart and soul are open to love.*

- *I know that money is energy; I create conditions for this energy to flow in my life.*

- *I sleep well, dream well, and wake feeling replenished.*

- *I Am guided by intuition and ancestral wisdom; I trust this guidance.*

- *I love my body; my body loves me.*

- *I Am enough. I see myself, and I Am enough.*

Affirmations for Artists

- *I Am doing the work that only I can do; I Am answering the call of my spirit.*

- *I Am my own creative expression. I honor my gifts, and I do not compare my work.*

- *I silence the noise of competition; I follow the sound of my own voice.*

- *I Am not afraid of grief. I use it in my work, and it becomes service.*

Affirmations for Organizers

- *I do not measure my reach against the need. I hold my position and do what is mine to do.*

- *I allow others to care for me.*

- *I practice daily joy. I bring joy to my work. I do not allow anyone to take my joy.*

- *Healing is vital to our movements. It expands our capacity to live.*

- *Yes, I do have time for intimacy, and I Am loved deeply.*

Affirmations for Healers, Holders, Practitioners

- *I honor boundaries. I respect the space between me and those I work with.*

- *I Am a guide, I Am a witness. I Am not the healing.*

- *I Am intentional with my own care. I honor the needs of my body, mind, and spirit.*

- *I Am comfortable saying no.*

- *I receive the energetic exchange of money for my work with ease, grace, and alacrity.*

- *I trust the capacity and body wisdom of my clients and those I work with.*

Affirmations for Pregnancy

- *I Am carrying the glory of my ancestors' dreams. We are loving our lineage forward.*

- *My body is home for your body. I Am grateful for you.*

- *I Am grateful for my wonderful body, which nurtures my healthy baby, I have all that I need to hold and birth new life.*

- *The sound of my beating heart lets you know you are loved.*

- *We are healing generational grief; my child knows they are loved, seen, cherished.*

- *You are not just of my body; you are of my heart, soul, and being.*

Affirmations for Parenting

- *I circle my child with love; they are visible only to love.*

- *I listen deeply to my children. I see them as whole and separate beings.*

- *I model self-love and care for my children.*

- *I create space for alone time to nurture my needs.*

- *I Am worthy of loving support. I ask and I receive.*

Affirmations for Educators

- *My work is my vocation. I love being an educator.*

- *I embrace the opportunity to teach and learn from my students.*

- *I see the student, not their story. I expect them to thrive.*

- *I embrace loving boundaries with my students. I trust their capacity to learn.*

Affirmations for Abortion

- *I release and let go of this pregnancy without fear or shame.*

- *I own and love my body, and I choose my life path.*

- *My choice today does not dictate my choice tomorrow.*

- *I receive, I bless, and I let go.*

- *My body is healthy, strong, and powerfully mine. I Am always at choice.*

- *I am grateful for the choice I made.*

Affirmations for Singlehood

- *I Am choosing to be my own partner.*

- *I enjoy being with myself.*

- *I love my own company; I decide when I share my time with others.*

- *I give myself the love I need.*

Closing

When you reach the sixteenth day of your practice, give yourself a half hour for reflection. Please consider these questions and record your answers in your journal:

- How do you feel?

- Was this practice of service to you?

- How?

- Which affirmations did you choose?

- Why?

- Have you noticed a shift in your personal narrative?

- What, if anything, is different?

You may choose to begin the fifteen-day ritual again with new affirmations. There is no closing to this practice; it can be ongoing, as you decide.

Beloved community, please write your own affirmations if you do not see what you need on our list. Also, feel welcome to tailor what you do see to suit your needs. Speak these words of love to yourself daily, and *be ye transformed by the renewing of your mind.* *Audio recordings of these practices are available at soundstrue.com/vibration-of-grace-bonus.

—————— Your Sacred Presence ——————
A 21-DAY PRACTICE

This offering is to be practiced over 21 days without interruption. If you miss a day, please go back to the beginning and start again. I understand that this practice may not be possible, as many of us have very full lives. Please read through the ritual and see if it will work for your present moment. If not, do return to this offering when it makes sense for you.

Each morning begins with meditation, affirmations, and toning. Each night before you sleep, you will journal, take a medicine bath or rinse, and practice visioning. For the morning practice, there are seven days of ritual that you will cycle over three weeks, repeating each practice three times (for example, the practice for days one, eight, and fifteen will be the day-one morning ritual). For the evening practice, you will journal and answer the same three questions nightly, take your bath or rinse, use the evening meditation that includes visioning, and then rest. We engage in this 21-day practice to regain clarity of purpose, to source and center our heart-led desires, and to reconnect with our power. This ritual will also clear energetic debris that can cling to us as we move through the world.

Tools

- a journal (may also be recorded)
- three medicine baths: one gallon of rosemary tea, bay leaf tea, rue leaf tea
- a timer with a soft ring

Preparation

Set an intention for this ritual. What do you hope to achieve? Consider this question and write the answer in your journal. Then, mark 21 days on your calendar and choose a date to start. If you are able, keep your practices to the same time every day. Begin your morning practice before you engage with work, computer, or phone. Close out your day with your evening practice—once you have finished work and silenced all devices.

You will be working with one medicine bath each week, one gallon of tea that may be prepared at the start of each week.

- **Rosemary tea for the first week** (prepare day 1): Boil a handful of fresh or dried rosemary sprigs in a gallon of water for about ten minutes; let tea sit and steep for at least three hours. The rosemary may remain in the tea.

- **Bay leaf tea for the second week** (prepare day 8): Boil a handful of fresh or dried bay leaves in a gallon of water for five minutes; let sit and steep for at least three hours. Remove bay leaves before using.

- **Rue leaf tea for the third week** (prepare day 15): Throw a handful of rue leaves into boiling water, adjust temperature to simmer for 15 minutes, and then let sit for at least three hours. Strain before using.

We will be going into bath rituals and recipes in more depth in the next chapter, but for now, just know that in this 21-day practice, you will use about two cups of tea for each daily rinse or bath.

Refrigerate the prepared tea bath; use as needed. If you are using it as a rinse, you may warm the tea before taking it into your shower.

Morning Ritual

Each morning when you wake, rise and go to where you will be practicing your meditation. Set a timer for thirty minutes. Open your ritual by saying a prayer, one from your tradition, and give thanks for another day of living. Honor the ancestors of the land supporting where you are, and honor the ancestors of your lineage, those who have come before and those who may follow. Begin your meditation. If you are sitting, sit comfortably with your back supported. If you prefer a standing meditation and it is available to you, stand and soften your knees with a slight bend, legs hip-width apart, and feel your feet planted on the floor. You will be swaying side to side, arms loose and hands at rest—or move your arms and hands slowly around your body if you wish. Once in position for meditation, close or soften your eyes by allowing your eyes to gaze downward. Bring your awareness to your breath. Inhale slowly through your nose and exhale audibly through your mouth; give this breath sound.

As you breathe, begin to journey around your body with your mind. Begin at the back of your neck and shoulders and make your way down your spine, vertebrae by vertebrae, as if you are descending or running your hands down the rungs of a ladder. Notice your sacrum, the backs of your thighs, knees, calves, the soles of your feet, and breathe deeply as you move your mind around your body. From the soles of your feet, you will then journey up your front body, your shins, knees, thighs, and then your torso, beginning with your perineum, pelvic floor, navel, stomach area, up between your breasts, the base of your throat, between your eyes, and the crown of your head. If you are standing and moving, you are breathing and noticing while swaying side to side; if you are seated, you are resting and allowing your body to be supported. Once you arrive at your crown, you are ready to begin your affirmation and toning practice. If the timer rings before you finish, keep going and complete the day's practice. If you finish before your timer sounds, sit or sway quietly until it does. Speak a few words of closing, by saying aloud that you are closing the space, sealing it shut, and give thanks for the opportunity to care for yourself. Speak your affirmation out loud to yourself throughout your day.

Days 1, 8, 15:

Affirmation: *I trust my body's wisdom; I believe myself.*
Tone: *Ahhhhhh*

Inhale deeply, exhale your affirmation; then inhale deeply, exhaling your tone. Choose a note that is comfortable and easy to tone. Repeat this practice five times.

Days 2, 9, 16:

Affirmation: *I hear and I know. I listen and I grow.*
Tone: *Ouuuuu*

Inhale deeply, exhale your affirmation; then inhale deeply, exhaling your tone. Choose a note that is comfortable and easy to tone. Repeat this practice five times.

Days 3, 10, 17:

Affirmation: *I see clearly and receive the guidance I need.*
Tone: *Eeeeee*

Inhale deeply, exhale your affirmation; then inhale deeply, exhaling your tone. Choose a note that is comfortable and easy to tone. Repeat this practice five times.

Days 4, 11, 18:

Affirmation: *I speak the word and it is so. I plant the seed
and let it grow.*
Tone: *Iiiiii*

Inhale deeply, exhale your affirmation; then inhale deeply, exhaling your tone. Choose a note that is comfortable and easy to tone. Repeat this practice five times.

Days 5, 12, 19:

Affirmation: *I feel truth at the center of my being; I trust what I feel.*
Tone: *Hummmmm*

Inhale deeply, exhale your affirmation; then inhale deeply, exhaling your tone. Choose a note that is comfortable and easy to tone. Repeat this practice five times.

Days 6, 13, 20:

Affirmation: *I am my word, my word is truth.*
Tone: *Ohhhhh*

Inhale deeply, exhale your affirmation; then inhale deeply, exhaling your tone. Choose a note that is comfortable and easy to tone. Repeat this practice five times.

Days 7, 14, 21:

Affirmation: *I Am a powerful being.*
Tone: *Yayyyyy*

Inhale deeply, exhale your affirmation; then inhale deeply, exhaling your tone. Choose a note that is comfortable and easy to tone. Repeat this practice five times.

Evening Ritual

Every night before bed, after you have silenced all devices for the day, prepare your tea for your bath or rinse, and sit down with your journal to write. The evening rituals will follow this format:

Each evening you will open your journal (or recording device) and answer these questions:

- Did you speak your affirmation to yourself throughout the day?

- How did this make you feel?

- How are you feeling now?

Record these questions and your answers and anything else that may be rising in your spirit. Then prepare your bath or take your warmed tea into the shower.

- days 1 through 7, rosemary tea bath

- days 8 through14, bay leaf bath

- days 15 through 21, rue leaf bath

If taking a bath, pour about two cups into a full tub of water; if taking the tea into the shower, pour some of it over your crown, your forehead area (also known as the third eye), the base of your throat, and the back of your neck. Let it spill over your shoulders and down your front and back body. Use your soap before pouring over your body; if in the tub, use soap sparingly.

When you're in bed, recall your intention for this 21-day practice. Close your eyes and bring your awareness to your breath. Inhale deeply through your nose and exhale slowly, softly and audibly through your mouth. Cycle this breath five times, noticing your back body as you breathe. Allow your neck to be supported where you lay. As you are able, please relax your shoulders, and move your awareness down your spine, vertebrae by vertebrae, to your sacrum, inhaling deeply through your nose and exhaling slowly and audibly through your mouth. Begin to imagine your intention realized. See yourself in your mind's eye; imagine yourself at ease. Guide your mind to visioning the way we guide children to task, with gentle persistence. See yourself inside of your dreams, not as if you are watching yourself but from a place of having already received the grace you are seeking.

Closing

When you wake on the morning of your 22nd day, after you do whatever your usual morning practices are (my daily practice is prayer, walking meditation, and then a good cup of coffee), find your way to your journal and notice how you are feeling. Write down any shifts in your perspective, epiphanies, ideas, new or old knowings—write it all down so that you have it for reference. Reflect on what was difficult about this ritual and also what may have become easier or harder as the days passed. Congratulate yourself for completing the ritual, and know that you may work with this 21-day practice as often as you wish. *Audio recordings of these practices are available at soundstrue.com/vibration-of-grace-bonus.

part two

CARETAKING
—— *the self* ——
HEALING HARM

once my heart was broken
i began to live the lie,
crawled into that tiny space where dreams go to die—
collected glass and weaponry that tiny hands can hold
built myself a room of steel, pretending to be bold
and I made some things, even bought some wings that wouldn't fly
there was so much more, behind every door, but who am I?

3

Sound to Release Grief:
Giving Us Free

experienced my first grief-letting circle when I was nine years old. The intergenerational gathering of Black women at my father's home church in Apalachicola, Florida, did not use the term "grief-letting"; they simply called it the "Women's Circle," and they met weekly at the church on Thursday evenings. I was part of the junior choir, and choir practice would happen while the women met behind closed doors. Almost every time, I would sneak out of choir practice and find my way to their circle, drawn by the sounds coming from the room.

Three years after my mother left us, my father moved me and my four siblings out of Brooklyn to his hometown of Apalachicola, Florida, hoping to have an easier life. My older sister and brother had dropped out of school; truancy laws in New York could have landed my father in prison. He thought a slower pace and the support of his large family would help get his children back on track. My father's people are Missionary Baptists, with Holy Roller praise woven throughout the ministry. As soon as we arrived, we were expected to be in church five days a week, and thrice on Sundays. My two older siblings rejected this outright and promptly found their way to local trouble. The younger two and I had to obey, and we did, mostly.

I loved being in church. I felt a sense of community and belonging. The singing and live music covered me in joyous sound. I didn't understand much of the doctrine; some of it was even scary to me. The language of homosexuality being an unforgivable sin was particularly frightening as I had several crushes on my female teachers and some of my girlfriends. I decided that the sermons were not about me, but the music, the dancing and shouting, the release I felt—*these* were wonderful. I was nine years old and living with the trauma of sexual abuse and abandonment. I was able to move some of this grief weekly in church because of the energy of praise. I jumped, shouted, and hollered with the rest of the congregants, and I felt lighter afterward, connected to something other than my fear.

During choir practice, I sat in the back of the room near the exit, and I would slip out as soon as the choir director turned his back. I would stand outside the door where the women were meeting and listen. I could hear voices humming and then someone's hum would become a moan. It sounded like moaning and singing at the same time and felt familiar to me. Grace had taught me how to hum and tone long musical notes to myself to help me sleep past nightmares, which I began to experience around the age of seven, terrible dreams about being in danger with no way to safety. Listening to the humming, I felt a kinship with these women, that we had something in common. I would slip into the room and sit in a corner trying to make myself small so they wouldn't notice me and send me back to the children's room. Of course, they noticed me.

After a bit, someone would begin to cry and then wail. The woman wailing would lay her head in another woman's lap, and that woman would begin to cry too. The elders, known as the mothers of the church, would rise and go to the younger women and lay hands on shoulders and touch the backs of necks, singing, sounding, and moaning into the body of the person they were tending. The woman receiving would cry with abandon, sometimes sobbing lying down on the floor. The moaning, humming, and sounding would continue, a chorus of voices; I could not separate one from the other. Often I would cry and hum too. After a while, the crying would come to quiet. There would be coughing and folks blowing their noses. Someone would laugh, and soon everyone was laughing and talking about being hungry and who brought what foods to share—pound cake, lemonade, fried fish, and other delicious things. I would quietly leave to go back to choir practice, feeling the joy the women were now sharing with each other.

Our time in Apalachicola, Florida, was brief. Six months after we arrived my aunties went to my father and asked him to gather his children and go back to New York. We were simply too wild, and there was nothing more they could do to support my father in raising his unruly children. We left the way we came, a two-day journey on a smelly Greyhound bus. I was the only one in my family who was sorry about leaving.

I felt the power of love inside the rituals I witnessed. Now when I hold healing circles, I remember the mothers of the church who allowed me to sit and be part of their weekly sessions, and I am forever grateful. They were my teachers, showing me what was possible.

Our Expressions of Grief, What Has Shaped Us

Dear family, take a moment to consider your relationship to grief. Please take a few deep, slow breaths by inhaling through your nose and exhaling audibly through your mouth. Then think about what happens in your body when you feel like crying. How does it impact you when someone is expressing grief in front of you or to you? How did your family of origin handle your expressions of grief?

In my home, I was told that if I did not toughen up the world was going to chew me up and spit me out. My father would tell us that if we didn't stop crying, he would give us something to cry about. My brothers were not allowed to express grief; they had to "man up." There was no one in my family and no one I knew growing up who was ever allowed or encouraged to cry. Even the youngest ones were told to "stop crying like a baby," and we did as we were told. We learned how to swallow and suppress our sadness. We learned how to *keep it moving*, to keep doing whatever task was in front of us regardless of how we were feeling or what care we needed.

Now, dear family, we know that there are horrific reasons for legacies of grief suppression. My father had terrible things happen to him as a boy, a Black child growing up in the south. He ran away from home when he was fourteen years old and found his way to New York City, thinking his life would be better there. When he told me to stop crying and toughen up, he was trying to protect me. My father died of a heart condition at 49 years old. His heart was clogged, blocked with the energy of unlet grief. When we continuously swallow our pain, it becomes lodged in the vital organs of the body, because the energy must go somewhere. In African and Indigenous spirituality, there are common rituals around energetic healing and the repurposing of grief. Albert Einstein declared what my ancestors knew, that energy can be changed from one form to another. We assure you that the energy of grief, when allowed expression, may be sourced to create systems of care. Grief can be powerful medicine once we change our relationship to grieving. Being present with our own grief and allowing it to move creates spaciousness in the body and a deeper capacity for living. When we are in our own practice of grief-letting, we can be present and witness others in their process.

Many of us have pain-filled stories of not being allowed to express our full feelings as children. These stories are important. Sometimes we get caught in our stories and don't move. We get stuck, circling old harms and narratives, and grief and trauma become fused together. They are not the same thing. Grief is an organic response to loss, frustration, longing—so many things can cause grief to rise. Trauma can be caused by physical, emotional, and mental abuse. We feel grief around trauma, but not all grief is traumatizing.

Sometimes we cling to the pain of our stories as a way of being in relationship with the past. Healing does not mean forgetting or dishonoring what we or our ancestors have endured. It means that we are more than the pain that gets stuck in our throat and dictates our choices. We can hold story and freedom from story, sourcing the power of memory while not allowing memory to anchor us to tragedy and horror.

My father is not to be blamed or shamed for not knowing how to caretake his or our emotional needs. He was taught by his father, and his father before, how to survive. *The Vibration of Grace* is about loving ourselves into new ways of being, healing generational grief, and creating holistic pathways for us, our children, and the children to come.

GRIEF-LETTING CIRCLES

This community ritual to shed grief creates the opportunity for witnessing, support, reflection, and connection. We suggest a circle of three or four people to start, and you are welcome to engage a two-person practice as well. The number of people may grow as you become more experienced with circle work. I have held in-person grief-letting circles with over a hundred people, and I've attended larger circles guided by our beloved ancestor and grief doula Sobonfu Somé. To be witnessed is powerful medicine and can break up narratives that drive us toward isolation. We experience in real time that we are not alone in our suffering. This ritual also helps us to practice normalizing feelings of sadness.

Tools

- a small table to build an altar and a treasured object to place there
- a time piece with a soft ring
- several boxes of tissue
- flowers (fresh if possible)
- water for drinking
- a prepared meal, to be enjoyed after the ritual
- bay leaf tea for a bath or rinse after the ritual
- journals and pens
- pillows and blankets
- comfortable clothing
- house music playlist or songs you love to dance to
- agreements

Preparation

If you decide to engage this ritual, think about who you wish to be in circle with. Sometimes it takes a moment to connect with folks who are available to engage with grief work. Once you identify those who will be in circle, invite them to a pre-ritual check in. This can be a phone call or a video chat where each person gets to reflect on the intention and agreements shared here, which will create the container for your time together.

Intention. The intention of this ritual is to be witnessed and held by the circle while connecting with your grief. This work is about creating the opportunity for inner movement, deeper understanding of what you may be holding, and what you wish to release. We do not circle to "fix" each other or solve each other's problems. There is so much care inside of simply witnessing and allowing the person in front of you to make their own discoveries.

Agreement: Stay with yourself. The first agreement is that you will stay with yourself. Staying with yourself means not interrupting another's process. During the ritual, each person will have 35 minutes to speak; no one has to use all the time, just what is needed. Everyone in the circle must agree to witness silently and be present without judgment. Do not contradict anything that is said during a person's share, even if they are berating themselves. Do not counter with any assurances of their beauty or power; let them be. If during the ritual someone begins to cry during their share, you may ask in the moment if that person wishes to be touched. If the answer is yes, and it is available to you, place a steady hand on their shoulder or upper back. If the answer is no, do not take it personally; let the person sharing dictate what they need.

The person sharing should agree to practice staying with themselves as well. If you are speaking about harm that has been done to you, speak about how it has impacted your life and what it has caused you to feel. Try not to speak about the person who did the harm; do not consider their motives. Stay with yourself.

Agreement: Keep it private. Agree that you will keep each other's stories private. You may share about your own experience with the grief circle, but you may not share another person's experience. And after you close the ritual, if you meet outside of your circle, you must have each other's permission to discuss anything that happened during circle time. Consider and discuss these agreements, and ask everyone if they have more agreements they would like to bring to the circle.

Before closing your check-in call, make sure that you have everyone's consent around the shared agreements. Then choose a date and time to gather. (I suggest an afternoon ritual.) Give yourselves at least four hours to be together. Each person should bring food and a non-alcoholic beverage to share. Alcohol will mask feelings, and it is important to stay present with whatever arises. Participants should bring an altar piece, something precious that they will take with them when you close the ritual, and a small bouquet of flowers. Also, people should bring a journal or something to write with, a pillow, and a blanket. You will be dancing together to close this ritual or choosing a movement that is accessible to all, so decide on a playlist that has a favorite song from each participant. I am an old "House Head" from way back. If you don't know what house music is, here is your invitation to research it. Everyone should dress comfortably. Silence all phones and devices during your time of practice, and do not use unless there is an accessibility need for note-taking. Write your agreements on a large sheet of paper that you will tape to a wall for everyone to see on the day of the ritual.

Medicine Bath (Bay Leaf) for gentle care. The night before you gather, everyone should prepare a bay leaf tea for the medicine bath or rinse to take after the ritual. Bay leaf is a gentle medicine that cleanses and soothes the energetic body. Boil a gallon of water and place a handful of bay leaves in the pot, turn off the boil, and let the water sit on the stove overnight and throughout the day. Again, this bath is to be taken once you return home after your grief-letting circle. Before using, remove the leaves if you will be taking the tea into the shower; if using in the bath, pour the entire contents into a full tub of water. For the shower, pour the tea slowly over the crown of your head, your throat, and the back of your neck, while standing under the flow of water. If using in a bath, pour the tea with the leaves into a full tub of water and sit and soak. If it is available to you, rub the leaves between your palms and inhale the fragrance. If you are able, lean back and submerge yourself. Gather the leaves after your bath and discard how you wish.

Ritual

Invite participants to arrive a half hour before you begin. The place you choose to gather can be the home of any circle member or any safe place where you will not be disturbed. Only circle participants should be present—no pets or other people. Pets are wonderful support but can distract us from the grief-letting process.

As folks arrive, co-create the space by choosing where you will sit and placing your pillow and blanket there. I like to sit on the floor; you may sit in chairs or on couches—just make sure you can face each other. Place the small table you have chosen for your altar close to your circle. Decorate the room with flowers. Each person should place their flowers where they can be seen or smelled, and save some for the altar. The flowers bring the energy of beauty to your gathering.

When ready, everyone takes their seat. Open your circle by revisiting your shared agreements and asking participants if there is anything anyone wishes to add. Then, honor the land that is supporting your ritual by acknowledging the first peoples who lived where you are now standing. Afterward, each person is invited to bring their chosen piece for the altar forward and share its significance before placing it on the altar. When the altar is complete, choose the order of sharing among yourselves and who will hold the timepiece first. Each person will have a turn to be a timekeeper, with this position changing between sharings. Once this is decided, you will begin a brief meditation.

Have the first timekeeper set the timer for *seven* minutes. Invite everyone to close or soften their eyes and to bring their focus to their breath. Begin a conscious breath practice: each person is to inhale deeply through the nose and exhale through the mouth as slowly as they can and to keep to their own pace. Bring full awareness to the breathing practice. If the mind guides you away from this task, gently guide yourself back to your breath.

Once the timer chimes, everyone should slowly bring themselves back to the circle and prepare for the first person's share. When the first person is ready to share, the timekeeper sets the timer to 35 minutes.

Sharing. It is probable that you have been preparing for this moment since your pre-ritual check-in call. You may be feeling fear or overwhelm or suddenly have no words. Be gentle with yourself and allow yourself any response. Do not feel pressured; there is no "right" way to share. Whatever you wish to say, be, or do with your time is what is needed by you at the moment. Perhaps begin your share with how you are feeling about sharing. Maybe there is something weighing on your spirit and you wish to speak of it in circle to hear it said out loud. I have sat in circles where the person sharing used all their time to cry, feeling the grace of loving witness. It is entirely up to you. If you cry, try to allow any sounds that accompany your tears, which helps the energy of grief release. Practice breathing deeply as you share, and be mindful not to rush through your words. When you hear the timer chime, begin to close your sharing. You do not have to end abruptly; note that you have heard the timer and close your time with as much ease as possible.

Witnessing. It's important to take care of yourself while witnessing. Sometimes when we give our attention to a person's share, we are moved by what is being said in ways that make it difficult for us to be present. If this happens, practice conscious breathing by guiding your awareness to inhaling through your nose and exhaling softly through your mouth. Remind yourself that you are safe and holding space for a friend. Practice staying with the present moment by listening to what is being said without allowing your mind to take you to your own experience. You will have time to share. As you witness, hold in your spirit the highest knowing of the person sharing. Breathe and know that your witnessing and regard are profound acts of love.

Journaling, Pause for ten minutes after each person's share. Have the new timekeeper set the timer. Use this time to journal, use the bathroom, get more water, stretch. Unless it is necessary for health, try not to eat anything, for eating will change the energy of what you are feeling. When journaling, stay with your feelings; do not try to decipher them in the moment. You may try freewriting by recording your thoughts as they pass through your mind. You may also try using these prompts as a guide:

- Was it difficult listening to this story? Why?

- Did you feel any discomfort in your body during the share?

- If yes, where?

- Do you feel any resistance to continuing this ritual?

- If you were the person who shared, how did this feel?

- How are you feeling now?

When the timer chimes, move slowly back into your posture of listening, reset the timer for 35 minutes, and invite the next person to share.

Closing

After each person has shared and journaled, it is time to close the ritual. Thank each other for bravery and presence, witnessing, humor, and grief. Together remember the agreements around privacy. Speak words that honor each other and the ancestors who walk beside each of you. Then, each person will remove their altar item and say a word of closing to seal the moment. When everyone has had their say, stand, stretch, hug if that is permissible and accessible to you, and get ready to move, dance, and eat. Turn on the shared playlist and move your bodies around the space. Then get yourselves a plate and sit and enjoy your meal.

Everyone is to take their flowers when they leave, and when they get home, take their prepared medicine bath or rinse, and rest well. After resting, return to journaling and revisit the time in circle. You may discover a new life practice waiting there for you, something that supports a deeper and truer expression of you.

Grace has told me that one day people will gather regularly to engage in grief-letting rituals. She says it will be as common as sitting around a table to play cards or share a meal. The circles will be as varied and as rich as our interconnected communities, and there will be a place for everyone who wishes to be part of the ritual.

Grief-Letting: Pulling, Wailing, Releasing Anger

The practice of pulling will teach you how to dislodge another person's energy from your body, wailing will help you give sound to the grief you have no words for, and the ritual we offer around releasing anger will support you in accessing and releasing this emotion. These rituals are tailored for solo practice, which gives you the opportunity to lean fully into all that you are feeling without managing or censoring yourself, the way we can do when others are present. You are also encouraged to share your grief-letting process with those you feel held and seen by, so that these folk can check on you as you learn how to work with these offerings.

Before we introduce this next set of rituals, we will share a synthesized story of people who came to practice with me over the last three years. Their stories have been synthesized to protect the identities of those involved (some whose names I never even knew). These rituals changed their lives.

They came to my virtual table over the summer of 2020, heavy with the weight of unlet grief. They were organizers and strategists, and they worked with several organizations on the front lines of social justice movements, formed to fight for body sovereignty, climate justice, and the Movement for Black Lives (M4BL). They were experiencing mental health challenges and found themselves incapacitated by the recent murder of George Floyd. It was also a time of global fear because of COVID-19, when many people were dying daily. These organizers and strategists kept trying to support the organizations they worked with, wanting to be of service to the moment of profound need. Demonstrations were happening around the world to protest George Floyd's murder, and they wanted to support these historic happenings.

When I meet with people, I am allowed to know their pronouns, whether they are parents, and whether they are partnered, and that is all. The less I know, the better channel I can be, and any information required for their healing is revealed as needed.

These activists came to me afraid, with a dwindling capacity to do anything they wished to do. I could see that grief was blocking their ability to think. They had always relied heavily on their intelligence and had lots of practice successfully identifying the anger and grief of others, but they had little to no experience accessing and moving their own grief and anger. The focus was always output, with very little inner scaffolding for their own internal needs and care. There was a conscious desire and commitment to save the world and an unconscious agreement that they would donate their lives to do it.

During our work together, they learned how to wail. Childhood trauma was part of the reason they wanted to be organizers. They are fighting for a world where all children are safe, and they learned that to be well they must also tend to the hurt children inside their own beings. The wailing practices allowed access to pain and grief they had no language for, only sound and tears. Some hurt predates language; our baby selves cannot talk about harm that can be accessed only by leaning into memories stored in the body. Because they could not consciously access the memories, they were surprised by how much grief they were carrying. They discovered that the body can release what the mind cannot or will not remember.

The profound grief felt from witnessing the murder of George Floyd is a normal response to terror. What happened with the activists and organizers who were working with me is that the terror became entwined with their personal experiences of heartache and emotional abuse, and they could not separate the two. Once they began to practice holding themselves, they were able to honor and release the grief they embodied from their work. Grief from the embodiment of generations of dehumanized Black people. Grief from organizing in their own communities. Grief from the summer of 2014 when Mike Brown was killed in Ferguson, Missouri. By 2020, Ahmaud Arbery, Breonna Taylor, George Floyd, Tony McDade, Asia Jynaé Foster, and so many more had been killed. The compounded grief from these times and before could no longer be contained or compartmentalized. This grief had to be moved so that they could acknowledge, access, and begin to heal the wounds of their childhood.

I am grateful to share that they are now doing and feeling quite well, no longer oversaturated by grief and unable to hear their own voices or identify the core of who they are. They can be with themselves while navigating the terrain of their vocations, responding to the call of their work as organizers, holders of holders. They began regular practices to move anger and also use the ritual of pulling to keep moving old hurt out of their bodies. They are keeping to the practices they created to allow grief to flow, and they prioritize their care as they continue to do their good works in the world.

———— Ritual ————
OF PULLING

The ritual of pulling is sometimes referred to as "cutting cords." It is an energetic practice where one physically pulls and releases the invisible emotional ties that connect us to people, harm, places—anything we wish to disengage. There are many ways to do this practice; I will share what Grace has taught me.

When we do this ritual, we extract the root of the energy, pull and discard the connecting hook, and then place love in the space we have cleared. We do not "cut" the cord because cutting can leave roots. Essentially, we are reclaiming spaces within our energetic body that someone or something else is occupying. This work is done by using your imagination, fueled by your desire for release and self-ownership. I have found this ritual to be deeply effective when going through any kind of breakup or difficult transition. Folks are usually surprised by the amount of energy they are carrying that does not belong to them. Pulling energetic cords frees the body of another's presence and creates opportunity for perspective and clarity. When we hold anything too close, we cannot see it properly. This ritual can gift us with an appropriate sense of distance and support us in creating stronger boundaries.

(Note: In some traditions, when you locate the cord that connects you to another, you are guided to send love through the cord to the other person. Dear family, I don't believe in sending love while pulling cords. I feel that we are pulling someone for a reason, and we must center our care and love for ourselves first. Pulling cords is not about what or who you are pulling; it is about reclaiming your body by evicting what does not belong—so keep your focus on you.)

Preparation

We borrow from chakra science to work with this ritual. The chakra system originated in India, where it is described in some of the oldest Hindu sacred texts, called the Vedas. Chakras (the word means "wheel" in Sanskrit) are the body's energy centers. In yogic philosophy, there are seven chakras in the human body that correspond with specific nerve bundles along the spine and certain internal organs.

Each chakra governs values, desires, behaviors and corresponds to a different life intention. The root chakra (the first chakra) is housed at the tip of the tailbone and is associated with the perineum (the space between the anus and genitals) and the pelvic floor. It corresponds with our sense of stability. The sacral chakra (the second chakra) is housed below the navel and is connected to creativity and sexuality. The solar-plexus chakra (the third chakra) lives in the stomach area and is connected to our self-confidence and will. The heart chakra (the fourth chakra) is housed at the center of our chest and is connected to our ability and capacity to show love. The throat chakra (the fifth chakra) rests at the base of our throat and is connected to self-expression and our ability to speak our truths. The third-eye chakra (the sixth chakra) is located between the eyes in the center of our head and is linked to perception, awareness, and intuition. And the crown chakra (the seventh chakra),which is housed at the top of the skull, governs our connection to spirit, wisdom, and universal consciousness.

This is a very short explanation of the chakras, which are an endless and brilliant mapping of the body. I encourage you to do your own research here. In addition to the chakras, auras are the invisible energy fields that surround all of life. Some people can see auras. I feel and hear this invisible energy.

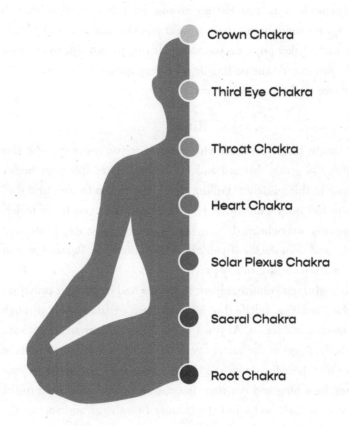

Crown Chakra

Third Eye Chakra

Throat Chakra

Heart Chakra

Solar Plexus Chakra

Sacral Chakra

Root Chakra

When we take in other people's energies, that energy will live inside of our chakras. The ritual of pulling removes this outside energy and creates a clear distinction between what belongs to us and what does not. Again, this ritual may be used to shift our connection to places, events, and people. Here we will focus on removing a person's energy from our body.

Decide whose energy you will be pulling. Work with one person at a time. Give yourself at least two hours to perform the ritual. Have a nourishing meal prepared for afterward, and do not eat an hour before the ritual. I recommend a quiet setting for this work. You will be listening to your inner voice or spoken words as you place affirmations in the spaces you clear. Find a comfortable place to lie down where you will not be disturbed. Resting on your back, have a pillow beneath your legs for support and space around you so that you can physically touch each chakra point on your body. If you are not able to use your hands, you may do the pulling in your imagination.

Silence all devices, and begin.

Ritual

Dear family, please check in with yourself as you move through this practice. Go gently forward and notice as you are able your body's response to this guidance. Pulling rituals can feel so freeing, and they can also feel quite difficult. If your body resists or you begin to feel emotionally overwhelmed, you may stop this practice. Pause and breathe and then decide if you are able to continue. Remember that you can always return to any practice.

To begin, rest comfortably on your back and begin your conscious breathing practice. Inhale through your nose, exhale audibly through your mouth, and repeat. As you are able, bring your awareness to your back body. Begin at the back of your skull and, vertebrae by vertebrae, guide your thoughts down the back of your neck and spine to your sacrum, breathing and noticing. Breathe and guide your mind to the end of your back body, and then slowly bring your noticing up the front of your body to the top of your skull. Continue to breathe deeply and evenly. Allow your body to be supported where you are resting, inhaling deeply and exhaling deeply with sound.

After you journey around your body with the breath, say these words out loud:

My body is my sanctuary, my body belongs to me.
I am circled by love, grace, and mercy.
I do this ritual now to release what does not belong to me,
To reclaim all of my body.
I am grateful for my body wisdom.
I am grateful for the presence and guidance of my ancestors.

(Please feel welcome to add your own language to this prayer as you feel led.)

Return to your breath practice, inhaling through your nose and exhaling through your mouth. When you are ready, begin to turn toward the person you will be pulling from your chakras. Lean into your memories; see them in your mind's eye. Recall what was wonderful about your connection and what was difficult or painful. Notice your breath, and keep to your practice of deep breathing as you stay with the memories that surface. See clearly who you will be evicting, and reach down to your root chakra to find the cord. Physically stretch out your arm and reach your hand to the space where your perineum lives; if this is not comfortable or available, please touch this space in your mind. Touch this part of your body, and imagine there is a cord sticking out, just enough for you to take hold of and begin to pull. Give the cord weight, color, and texture, and imagine that as you pull the cord, it is unraveling and leaving your root chakra. Pull and remember, pull and imagine, pull and allow the energy to leave. When the cord goes taut or you begin to cycle through the same memory, it is time to remove the hook. Imagine you are gently extracting a hook from your root chakra, much like removing a hook from a fish. If you are able, physically remove the hook, gather the cord that is attached to the hook, and toss it far away from your body. You may also do this ritual by visioning: see yourself remove the hook and gather and toss it far from your body.

Imagine that this energy will be repurposed. See it disintegrate and float out of the room like particles of dust to be gathered by the wind and taken elsewhere. Then return to the space you have cleared, and say your name out loud. Imagine filling your root chakra with your name and words that remind you of your power and worthiness. See your own root, like roots from a tree, moving from your body to the earth beneath your dwelling. Feel the certainty of anchoring, of being supported by the ground. Affirm that your root chakra belongs to you. Breathe deeply, and notice how you feel. Continue to affirm and breathe and vision yourself being held by your own words, voice, and intention.

You will then continue to move along your chakra body (from the root to the crown) to repeat the ritual. Each time remember the grace and challenge of the connection you are releasing and then reach in and pull the cord, evicting the energy and placing yourself, your word, in the space you have freed. You may find that each chakra is holding different things. Sometimes the cord will feel super long; other times, not. Often my clients find that the cord in the throat chakra is longest because of all that was left unsaid. Once you complete the crown chakra, it is time to close the ritual.

Closing

While inhaling deeply through your nose and exhaling through your mouth, take another journey around your body. Notice. Check in with yourself. How are you feeling? You can place one hand on your chest and one hand just below your stomach. Breathe deeply and be with yourself. Feel yourself supported where you are laying. When you exhale, be conscious of releasing all the air in your body and allow your body to relax.

When you feel ready, say or think these words:

> I close this ritual of pulling cords.
> I am wholly and fully myself.
> My body is my sanctuary; my body belongs to me.
> I Am (say your name here), and my body belongs to me.

Then, slowly rise, hydrate well with fresh water, and enjoy your meal. I encourage you to journal about your experience and findings.

This ritual can bring all the feels, tears, anger, laughter, and sometimes no feelings surface. It is particular to the release your body is needing. Be gentle, easy, and loving with yourself. Give yourself time to rest. After a few days, you should notice a feeling of spaciousness when you think of the person you've released. Usually, one ritual of pulling is all that is needed, although once I had to pull cords for a person several times. You will know by the way you feel when you think of the person.

You may engage this ritual as often as you wish, with at least three days in between each pulling. Listen closely to your body and be guided. *Audio recordings of these practices are available at soundstrue.com/vibration-of-grace-bonus.

—————— Ritual ——————
OF WAILING

The mothers of my church in Apalachicola, Florida, taught me about the powerful release that wailing can give us. Wailing is crying or expressing grief with sound as loudly or intensely as you are able. Many of the people I work with are not able to cry when they come to my table. I hear the same story often, that as soon as grief begins to rise, the mind steps forward with narratives about being "too blessed to be stressed" or too privileged to be expressing grief. They find themselves comparing their lives to the lives of people they consider less fortunate and decide that they do not deserve to grieve. Dear family, this is a lie and a profound disservice to the body. Swallowing grief does not improve conditions for anyone. In grief doula work, I have witnessed the triumphant release of this untruth again and again, and it is glorious to behold.

When we have a flesh wound, the body can heal once the wound has been tended to, as the flesh wants to knit together and become whole once more. It is the same with our spirit. We will not heal well if we do not tend to emotional harm and remove the blockages that come from not accessing full expression. Wailing takes us to the center of sorrow and gives it a way out.

Tools

- tissues or several handkerchiefs

- comfortable clothes

- a soft blanket and pillow

- water to drink

- a prepared meal

- a prepared medicine bath

- a journal

- a movie or song that evokes feelings of sadness

Preparation

Prepare a nourishing meal that you will enjoy after you complete this ritual. Please choose and prepare your medicine bath from our list of bath offerings. Find a movie or a song that moves you to tears. If you choose a song, create a playlist that has the song on repeat for at least an hour. Choose something that you feel a kinship with and that has an ending that leads to joy or the possibility of joy and a new day. For me, it is the movie *The Color Purple*. The last twenty minutes of *The Color Purple* brings me to tears every single time I watch the scene where Miss Celie sees her sister Nettie after thirty years of forced separation. Their reunion is a beautiful and moving moment that always leaves me sobbing as the credits roll. Longing for beloveds is a universal feeling, and I am reminded of how much I miss my mother, who died in 2014. These days, if I feel the weight of grief in my body and I am having a difficult time moving it, I will fast forward to the end of this brilliant story, and my body will release what it has been holding.

Grief just wants to be expressed; the body does not care why. Once we allow grief to flow, the tears that have been caught in the body move. As we deepen our practice of allowing this expression, we will be able to turn toward our personal stories. Crying for someone else's story allows the body to let go before the mind's habit reroutes the moment.

Often, people will tell me they are afraid that once they start to cry, they will not be able to stop. In all my many years of working with people around grief, this has never happened. Sometimes after this ritual, you may find yourself crying about any emotional shift, from diaper commercials to disagreements with a partner or colleague—this too passes. Once opened, you may find lots of things waiting to be held in your hands and grieved. Think of it as a good clearing for your psyche, and know that you do not have to do this work alone. If you can, let your friends and family know that you are going to be working with rituals to release grief and ask them to check on you. Be specific with your ask: give days and timing around calls and texts, and set the container for your care.

Ritual

Settle your comfortably dressed body in your favorite place to sit and rest. With your blanket and pillow, tuck yourself in and lean back. Have your tissues, water, and journal nearby, and limit distractions from devices. Please write down the answers to these questions:

- What is your relationship to crying?
- What happens in your body when you think about wailing?
- Are you feeling any fear? If yes, do you know why?
- What do you wish to receive from this ritual?

After you close your journal, please lean back and allow where you are resting to support the full weight of your body. Soften or close your eyes for a moment as you inhale deeply through your nose and exhale slowly and audibly through your mouth. Cycle this breath *five* times.

Begin watching the movie or listening to the song you have chosen. Allow yourself to lean into any grief that rises in your body, like nobody is watching—because nobody is watching. If you are able, let yourself make sound; give voice to your tears. Do not force yourself.

If you need to pause, stop your song or movie and turn your focus back to your breath, inhaling deeply through your nose and exhaling slowly through your mouth. Decide that you are crying for the characters on screen or the lyrics in the song; this might help your body relax. If you begin to cry and you are able, try humming. Hum, and allow your body to move with the sound of your voice. That could be swaying back and forth, or you may decide to walk around the room or lie down. Let your body guide the movement. Hum and cry with sound, and stay with your feelings. Let the energy run its course and flow as it needs to. A good, loud cry with mucus flowing and red, puffy eyes—let it happen.

Closing

When your grief begins to subside, drink some water, and when you feel ready, enjoy some of your meal. It is likely that your tears will exhaust you, and you will find your way to a good nap. When you wake, take a medicine bath or a shower, and prepare to journal. Please write down your answers to these questions:

- How do you feel?
- Were you able to wail?
- Did any memories come to your mind during the ritual?
- How did this ritual serve you?

After you journal, please decide that you will move forward slowly and gently. You may feel lightheaded after you close. Grief is weighty, and when it is released, it is like taking heavy rocks out of your pockets, rocks that you may have been carrying for a long time. Who are you without this weight? Give yourself a few days to settle into and integrate this new lightness of being. We invite you to practice wailing as needed. *Audio recordings of these practices are available at soundstrue.com/vibration-of-grace-bonus.

—————————— Ritual ——————————
FOR MOVING ANGER

Anger and grief are closely related, and often we mistake one for the other. Because anger can feel empowering and feeling sad can cause us to feel exposed and vulnerable, many of us will lead with anger when we are grieving. But anger is not sustainable. It peters out and leaves us depleted, and often regretful. When we avoid sadness, the anger that comes through us is often disproportionate to the circumstances we face. We end up dumping all the unlet anger we have been holding onto someone who does not deserve to receive the vitriol and venom. Anger is an important emotion. It is often the way the body communicates the trespassing of our personal boundaries. Anger is the body inviting us to listen and act.

When we don't know how to address our anger, the suppressed energy can become rage. Rage is excessive anger that can lead to violence against ourselves and others. Grace tells me that prolonged exposure to rage can also harm the internal organs. We feel that moving rage requires the presence of a learned healer, practitioner, or therapist because rage can be difficult to uproot on your own.

Please read through the following ritual and imagine yourself engaging with the practices. Notice your body's response. If you feel hopeful and interested, I believe the ritual for moving anger will serve you. If the ritual feels daunting, please trust your mind-body wisdom and consider having support for this practice. You can always return to any ritual. Often, a different day can yield a different response.

Here are rituals that will help you to move anger.

Tools

- 8 plates
- 2 pillowcases
- a hammer
- bay leaf bath

- chamomile tea

- rose petal tea

- rose water, essence of rose petals, or Florida water
  (a citrus-based cologne used to clear stagnant energy)

- a soft punching bag (can be a child's toy)

Preparation

You can go to Goodwill or any Dollar Store to purchase plates and pillow cases. Choose a pattern or a color you would never use at home. You can also use any of your old plates that you no longer want for this practice.

Prepare your bay leaf bath and a pot of chamomile-and-rose-petal tea. For the tea, you can use loose herbs (1 tablespoon of each herb in 2 cups of boiling water) or combine teabags. Let the tea steep, and add sweetener to taste (I suggest local honey). After the ritual, you will enjoy your tea while taking your bay leaf bath.

You will need to locate a place for this ritual where you will have some privacy: a room in your home (not your bedroom), backyard, driveway, basement, a park, near a river, somewhere where you will feel comfortable and safe. You will be hammering old plates and making some loud sounds, so choose a place where you will not feel self-conscious.

Before you move into the ritual, sit quietly for a moment with your journal. Gather yourself by bringing your awareness to your breath, inhaling deeply through your nose and exhaling audibly through your mouth. Please write down or record your answers to these questions:

- How do you generally respond when you are angry?

- What does anger feel like in your body?

- How was anger processed in your home when you were
  a child?

- Were you allowed to express anger?

As you journal, breathe deeply, consider these questions, and notice your body's response. Please write down your noticings in your journal, along with anything else you wish to record. When you are ready, set your own intention for this ritual or use mine: *To move anger out of my body; to connect with underlying grief.* Affirm this intention out loud to yourself several times, and then begin the ritual.

Ritual

Place one pillowcase inside of the other, and then place three plates inside the double-lined pillowcase and knot the end of it. Take the pillowcase full of plates and your hammer to the chosen location. Set these things down, and find your most comfortable position for breath practice, whether standing, sitting, or swaying from side to side. Bring your awareness to inhaling deeply through your nose and exhaling audibly through your mouth, and repeat this for a few minutes. As you breathe, consider all that you are feeling angry about, and know that during this practice, more things may surface. Decide that you will not check your feelings with logic or reason. You will allow yourself to be angry, and you will not harm your body—you are pounding plates, not yourself.

When you feel ready, take your hammer and begin to pound the plates as you hold your angry thoughts in your mind. Smash the plates to bits. Allow the anger you are feeling to lead this ritual. Make sure to engage your voice. Speak into what you are doing and allow yourself to say any words that need be said. Sometimes unresolved conflict will find its way to this moment; hammer away. Sometimes it is injustice you may feel helpless to change; hammer away. Often you are releasing anger around someone who harmed you. Once the plates have lost all shape and have become more like dust, check in with yourself. You may have exhausted the rage and found your way to grieving. But if you feel you need to, open the pillowcase and add more plates. Once you do find your way through anger to grief, allow yourself to cry, moan, lament. If you feel grief and have trouble allowing yourself to embody this feeling, please try the ritual for wailing. If you've used all your plates and still feeling angry, get into a cool shower, and under the running water, pour a bit of rose water or Florida water on the back of your neck and the base of your throat. The feeling should pass.

Another practice to move anger out of the body uses a punching bag. It can be something that you inflate, a child's toy, or a more substantial, soft bag that you can also kick. Again, be careful with your body; do not harm yourself. I have an inflatable bag that I punch when I'm feeling frustrated. Lately, I've been using the punching bag daily to release my anger and fear around the ever growing presence of fascist ideology and governing in my country and around the world. I move this energy out of my body, which helps to clear my mind, and then I know how best to direct my power to combat this threat to our democracy.

When working with this ritual you may begin to make connections between what causes you to feel anger; you may see a pattern to your behavior, the choices you make, and the situations and people you are drawn to. These patterns are often connected to our younger selves, where we may be caught recreating scenarios, sometimes to confirm a core belief about our worthiness and deservedness. We will speak more about this in our next chapter when we move through the ritual of soul retrieval.

Closing

When you have completed your ritual, take your bay leaf tea bath or rinse, warm your chamomile and rose tea, and drink your tea as you journal about the ritual and what you discovered. Please write down your answers to these questions:

- How are you feeling?
- Were you able to move anger out of your body?
- Did any memories surface for you during this ritual?
- What did you learn about yourself while engaging in this ritual?

Check in with your body, notice how you are feeling and what care you may need. Enjoy the meal you have prepared, and acknowledge that you are doing difficult and important work with yourself, for yourself.

Remember to be gentle with your body as you move through all the rituals to release grief and anger. The work of release is for your care; be as kind to yourself as you are with those you love. And take your time. Tune into the needs of your body. There is no rush.

4

Sound and Soul Retrieval: Gathering All of Yourself

Dear family, soul retrieval is a ritual in which you journey to past happenings of harm to take yourself out of the moment and give yourself the care, protection, and love you need to heal. We store unreleased fear in the body. Chronic pain, cyclical migraines, digestive issues, insomnia, health challenges with your blood, heart, liver, lungs, kidneys: these are all evidence of this truth. Grace says that pain and illness can be traced to violence, whether from our personal walk, ancestral trauma, or both. Soul retrieval is one way to disrupt, release, and repurpose the energy of violence. To work with this ritual, we surrender any notion of a "quick fix" and instead fully embrace the wisdom of practice. I have come to understand that healing can be a lifelong walk, and daily practice is an offering for the grace of being embodied.

The work of soul retrieval happens in the invisible imaginal realm. Consider that we work daily with things we cannot see yet have experiential evidence of, like radio waves, sound waves, and Wi-Fi. When we speak to each other, we are exchanging waves of sound. Most people cannot see energetic vibration, but we feel it. When engaging the ritual of soul retrieval, we venture beyond the world of tangible matter and turn toward the evidence of things not seen.

Rituals of soul retrieval are usually connected to shamanic practice. Shamanism is rooted in Indigenous and tribal cultures. Through trance work and plant-medicine journeys, shamans seek to bring the medicine of the spirit world to the physical world for guidance and healing. You do not need to be a shaman to practice this ritual with yourself. You *will* need to read carefully through the instructions, follow our guidance, and listen closely to your own wisdom. Soul retrieval rituals will often lead you to your younger selves, which provides an opportunity to heal the beginning place of you, to nurture and strengthen the root of you, and to replace narratives of self-loathing with mantras of worthiness. You become your healer.

Many of us have been taught to look to the horizon for a savior, that our salvation will come from someone or something outside of us. This walk to true freedom, however, requires that you do your part. You are the one who decides, who reaches for or accepts the hand extended, who takes the first step toward the life you desire. You have deeply rooted wisdom that lives within you, and though there are many brilliant healers, teachers, seers, medicine workers, and guides who can support you in finding your way to yourself, ultimately, it is your inner knowing and the sound of your own voice that will govern your life.

And dear family, unless you are a learned practitioner, *please do not try to guide anyone other than yourself through the ritual of soul retrieval.* I am grateful to witness so many people offering energy healing and holding. The desire to be of service comes from a place of love, I know. Yet there are some rituals that require us to study and practice for many years before we can safely guide others into invisible realms. Please reference our resource guide for masterful practitioners if you wish to have support for this practice.

Rituals of healing can be difficult work, and they can bring the sweetest, most surprising results. Imagine moving for days across a seemingly endless desert and then coming upon an oasis of fresh water with a field of yellow flowers blooming nearby where you get to drink long and roll around in fragrant beauty. This is how a soul retrieval practice can feel—profound effort for sweet rest and a deep sense of gratitude.

My Personal Walk

Through soul retrieval rituals, I was able to stop reliving trauma. My cyclical walk of dysfunctional relationships with partners, work, money, friendships, and housing began to shift when I turned toward my baby-girl selves and started loving them forward. I have returned to the doorstep where my mother abandoned me, and I have brought six-year-old gina home. I have rescued my five-year-old self, taking her out of the horror of being molested repeatedly by an older cousin. I have taken twelve-year-old gina in my arms and told her the truth about her beauty and capacity, and I have guided my thirty-five-year-old self through the practice of forgiving my father for his heinous acts of trespass.

I have witnessed the joy this ritual has brought to those I work with, as they revel in the realization that they are so much more than the abuse they endured. Fierceness, faith, wonder, and curiosity—the magic that children embody so easily—can return when we recover ourselves. And when we are no longer stuck in the past, we remember the dreams we dreamt when we believed we could do anything.

When Do I Practice? How Often?

When I began to work with soul retrieval, I would sit with this ritual three times a week, just before dawn. Generally, I rise at 5:00 a.m., when my home and the world around me feel most quiet. I started with a month of practice, which felt like a promise to myself that I could keep. Unlike the 21-Day Practice, there is not a set number of days or times you should practice soul retrieval rituals. It is a particular and personal walk dictated by what a person needs and has capacity for. And so, you decide how you wish to explore, how much time you will give to yourself, and when. Follow my example or create your own rhythm. Choose a time when you will not be disturbed. Once you begin, it is best to complete the journey and then close your ritual. Do give yourself time to settle and be with this medicine. Give this offering an opportunity to serve you.

And, sometimes there are simply not enough hours in your day. I remember how it felt to try to care for myself with a new baby. I barely had time to finish a cup of coffee. Doing anything outside of mothering my daughter was almost impossible. We know this is true for many caregivers and holders of spaces.

You can create a shorter version of this ritual of calling yourself home. After reading through the instructions, write a brief outline in your journal of what resonated for you, what parts feel like they may serve you. When you have a bit of space in your day, return to your outline to consider what you have written. You will know if there is any part of it you can engage in shorter increments—like imagining your younger self beside you at different times in your day while you tell them about your life now or speaking words of appreciation and love to your younger self as you work, eat, and rest. These practices do not require you to sit for long periods of time.

When you do begin working with this ritual, please do not rush through this good and powerful work. Please know that there can be immediate wins while some things may take longer to heal. If this feels like a burden, we encourage you to practice changing your mind. Speak these words to yourself out loud daily, as often as you wish, "I deserve the time this work requires. I create space for my healing."

How Old Is the One in Need? At What Age Shall I Begin?

If you have access to your memories, be guided by what reaches for you when you decide to do this work. Your body will tell you. Pay attention to your dreams, repetitive thoughts, your senses. One moment in time will stand out, and that is the age of the young one you will begin working with. If you do not have access to memory, sit with this question to begin the ritual: *Who wants to be heard?* Then listen and be guided. Make sure you hold space with one memory at a time, as you may be called to multiple moments of harm. Tell yourself that you have time to do this work and that all parts of you will get to be seen, witnessed, and loved by you.

During the ritual, you will address the younger versions of you as they know themselves, and not as the present-moment you. My five-year-old self is an innocent, who had barely left her Brooklyn neighborhood, whose whole world was her family and the people she knew from the block she lived on. At five she was already filling the position of caregiver and empath in her home, trying to soothe her siblings and parents by singing for them, seeking to absorb their grief so that they would feel better and she could feel safe, seen, and loved. When I speak with this baby girl, I reference the world she understands. I keep my tone gentle and my language simple.

When you begin to work with your younger selves, remember them. Who were they? How were they shaped by their position in the family as eldest, youngest, middle, or only child? Did they have a family name or nickname? If yes, address them this way. How was your younger self socialized regarding gender? Did this socialization feel good and true in your younger self's body? I did healing work with a trans woman whose soul retrieval practice centers on a child self who thinks of themselves as male and female. When she was quite young, she told her parents that she knew she was a girl. Her father's response to her knowing was violent and resistant, while her mother stood quietly by and said nothing. Her love for her parents and her desire to be loved by them forced her to comply with her father's demands to negate herself and embody his version of masculinity. When she returns to those harm-filled happenings with her parents to retrieve her child self, she uses the name and imposed identity her younger self tried to be. In doing so, she feels she is healing her relationship with the parts of her that tried to please her family. In this way, she is doing the work of loving herself into full integration of all of her being. This is her choice and her story.

As you read through the following soul retrieval ritual, listen to **your** body and notice **your** feelings. If you feel you can do this practice on your own, I believe you. If you feel you need support, I believe you. Asking for what we need is a practice too. Please be in this practice as you love yourself forward. Again, you may find information on healing arts practitioners in our resources section.

SOUL RETRIEVAL

———————— Ritual ————————

As you begin to gather tools for this ritual and move through preparing your meal, bath, and the space where you will practice, choose a prayer or poem that gives you a sense of ease and recite it softly to yourself. You may also listen to a recorded version. This can be a prayer that you create, one you choose from how you worship, or a poem that carries a vibration of possibility and grace. Lucille Clifton's "blessing the boats," is one of my favorite poems, alongside poems from Mary Oliver and Mirabai. Lean into the sound and feel the power and beauty of the language.

Tools

- a journal or recording device
- a timepiece with a soft-sounding alarm
- a prepared meal
- crystals, stones, and incense, if you like
- two prepared medicine baths (ingredients and recipes below)

Preparation

Plan to gift yourself at least two hours to complete the ritual. This time will include a healthy and grounding meal, a shower or a bath, and space to journal or record what you wish to remember. Once you become more practiced, you will be able to devote less time.

Prepare the day before or the day of your ritual by taking a medicine bath. You will be taking two baths, one before the ritual and one afterward. I've included some simple recipes here for you to choose the bath that best aligns with your needs of the moment. These medicine baths support the movement of energy that may be uncovered by this ritual. The combination of water, herbs, salts, essential oils, and intention helps us to feel lighter and clearer. Please be mindful as you prepare; be careful when working with boiling water for the teas.

These baths may also be used as a rinse in the shower. Prepare the mixture inside of a big pot, bring it to room temperature, take into the shower, and then use your hands to gather the medicine and pour it over the crown of your head, shoulders, the back of your neck, the base of your throat—let yourself be guided.

(There are prepared baths, created by learned practitioners, designed and rooted in their spiritual traditions. They are deep medicines, full of prayer, wisdom, spirit, and other ingredients that are sacred, but not mine to share. You can find some of these practitioners at the end of this book in the resources section.)

Medicine Bath to Release Grief: One cup of baking soda, one cup of sea salt, a few drops of lavender or rose essential oil. Sit in this bath as long as you can; allow yourself to rest.

Medicine Bath to Release Fear: Ruta graveolens or rue is known as the herb of Grace and thought to keep away evil spirits and to remind you of your divinity. I work with rue often, as I have found it to be a most generous and healing herb, great for dispelling narratives around fear. Rue is a plant that grows throughout the world. I have it in my garden, and I have seen growing wild rue in California and North Carolina. Rue can also be found and ordered online.

Find fresh or dried rue leaf. Boil a gallon of water for five minutes, then turn off the stove and place a handful of rue leaves into the water. Let this sit for a few hours. This tea can sit on your stove overnight if you use it the next day. If not, store it in the refrigerator, where it will keep for up to three days. Strain the tea before using it. This recipe is for two baths, so use half of the mixture. If you are using it as a rinse, pour the tea slowly over your crown and then allow it to spill over the back of your neck. Also pour some over the base of your throat and your front body. If taking a bath, sit in the rue bath for a half hour at most.

Medicine Bath to Clear Confusion: Place six teaspoons of ground nutmeg inside a tea bag or a coffee filter or a mesh type bag that can be sealed. If you are taking the tea into the shower, steep the filter in a gallon of boiled water for at least an hour. In the shower, pour all of the tea over your crown and the rest of your body. If you are taking a bath, place the bag in a full tub of water and sit in your tub for at least a half hour. You may hold the bag in your hands and inhale the scent if you wish. When you are done with your bath, simply discard the tea bag.

Medicine Bath to Release Listlessness: Add five cups of strong black coffee to a bathtub full of water, and rest in the water, up to your neck if you can. Stay in this bath for at least twenty minutes. I recommend not using this bath as a rinse in the shower—but if you do bring it into the shower, allow the coffee to cool first. Then pour over the back of your neck and the base of your throat, over your shoulders and solar plexus, your pelvic floor, your sacrum, and your feet.

Medicine Bath for Clearing Your Auric Field: Add seven white or pink carnation heads to a full tub of water. If you are not able to locate carnations, poms will work well too. Hold one flower head against each chakra, beginning at the root, and then on to your sacral, solar plexus, heart, throat, third eye, and crown chakras. Imagine and vision each flower absorbing energy from your chakra and clearing that center of what you do not need. As you move from your root chakra to your crown chakra, use a fresh flower each time and drop the used flower over the side of the bathtub. Have a paper bag ready to receive the flower. When you are done, close the bag and discard; do not touch the flowers again.

Medicine Bath for Deeper Rest: Place one handful of fresh or dried rosemary sprigs into one quart of boiling water, and boil for seven minutes. Let the rosemary tea sit on your stove for a few hours, and then strain. Pour all of the tea into a full tub of water, or you may use it as a rinse in the shower, slowly pouring it over your crown and the rest of your body.

While you are preparing and taking your bath, keep your mind with your body and stay with your feelings. If you have a prayer, song, mantra, or poem that calls to you, say or sing it to yourself. I encourage you to be with the sound of your breath and your voice—no music or other sounds while bathing. Just be with the sound of the water and the sound you create. Record or journal after your bath any thoughts or memories that may have come to your mind. As you move forward, all information revealed to you about you will serve your practice of dominion.

Ritual

You have completed all your ritual preparation, and you are ready to begin. Sit comfortably in a chair or on any soft surface that provides support for your back. Create a space in front of you that is level with where you are sitting, where you will invite your younger self to sit. Then close or soften your eyes and begin a conscious breath practice.

Notice your breath, and breathe intentionally. Inhale deeply through your nose and exhale through your mouth. Find your rhythm as you cycle this breath. Slowly bring your awareness to your body. As you are able, notice the back of your neck. Inhale through your nose, and as you exhale through your mouth, move your awareness slowly down your neck, past your shoulders, down your spine, vertebrae by vertebrae, to your sacrum. Inhaling slowly through your nose and exhaling through your mouth, notice your body. Move past your sacrum to where your perineum meets the chair, then notice the backs of your thighs, calves, ankles, and the soles of your feet. Breathe and notice. Breathe and notice. Then bring your awareness up the front of your body, past your shins, your knees, thighs, navel, the center of your chest, to the base of your throat, the space between your eyes, over your forehead, and to your crown.

Inhaling deeply through your nose, then exhaling through your mouth, begin to say this mantra out loud in between breaths:

> *My body is my sanctuary, and I am always home.*
> (Inhaling and exhaling)
> *My body is my sanctuary, and I am always home.*
> (Inhaling and exhaling)
> *My body is my sanctuary, and I am always home.*

Cycle this mantra. Focus on your voice, and listen to yourself. Take your time as you find your rhythm. When you feel ready, open your journal to write these agreements and your intentions for your ritual:

I Agree that my adult self will stay present.

Witness your grown hands holding the pen you write with and you who bought this book and decided to explore this modality and all the other grown-up things you handle and hold during the course of a day.

I Agree that I will allow any feelings that surface to move through my body.

If you feel like crying, you will let it happen.

I Agree that when the timer I set chimes, I will bring the ritual to a close.

This is a very important boundary; please acknowledge and agree.

The prayer you have been repeating for clarity will help you with the following questions; please write your answers in your journal:

- What do you wish to achieve?

- How do you want to feel?

- How will you care for yourself after you close?

When you are done writing, close your journal and place it within reach. Set your timer for 45 minutes. Return to your conscious breathing practice: inhaling through your nose and exhaling through your mouth. Lean back, allow the chair to support your weight, and stay with your breathing. Repeat softly, *my body is my sanctuary and I am always home*, and feel your body relax.

When you feel ready, and not before, begin to remember the you who has come forward to be held. See this you in your mind and invite her/him/us/them, or whatever pronoun feels right to you, into the room. Imagine and remember them; call them to you and invite them to the space you have prepared in front of you. Once you are sitting in front of your younger self, begin to speak to them with a calm voice. Tell your younger self that you will listen to anything they wish to share. Let them know that you will not interrupt because you are interested in what they have to say. Tell them that you have set a timer and that all the time that passes before the timer chimes belongs to them.

Return to your breathing practice, inhaling through your nose, exhaling through your mouth, listening to your breath, and noticing how you are feeling. If you feel embarrassed, ridiculous, or ashamed, simply notice. Be kind to yourself. Remind yourself that you are trying something new. Your conscious breath practice will help you to stay with whatever the younger you may have to say.

Notice the imagery that comes to your mind, the people, places, things, but don't try to make sense of anything just yet. Practice being present. Sometimes the moment is very clear, and you are taken to a familiar time. Do not push yourself to have a memory. Breathe and witness and listen. Allow feelings to surface and stay with yourself; try not to turn away. You are the adult in the room, holding space with them. Let your inner child speak and have their feelings; you practice listening and allowing your younger self to be the center of your attention and heard. Resist any urge to counter narratives that rise to mind. Often we will cover a painful memory with, "They did the best they could." This ritual is not about vilifying our loved ones who raised us, and it is not about forcing a sense of forgiveness for any harm done before we heal the wound the harm caused. Practice curiosity, as if you are hearing a story for the first time, because you are. The perspective of your child self will be very different from your present moment of adulthood. If resistance persists, try pretending that you are speaking with a child you have never met before, and listen.

Closing

When the timer chimes, know that it is time to close. Gather yourself by using your breath practice and mantra: *my body is my sanctuary, and I am always home.* Thank your younger self for coming and sharing. Tell them that you are closing the space and will return soon. Tell them that you appreciate all that they went through to keep you safe. Thank them for their bravery and for being so smart. Invite them to stay close to you, and tell them that you will take care of them. Give them appropriate boundaries. Tell them that there will be lots of opportunities to enjoy tasty treats, play, laughter, and age-appropriate things.

And tell them you will do all the adult work of parenting, managing money, partnerships, and all adult decisions. Then consciously close the moment by affirming out loud and with clear intention that your ritual of soul retrieval is closed, sealed until you decide to open the space again. Record your experience in your journal, take your medicine bath or shower, have a good grounding meal, and move slowly into your day. *Audio recordings of these practices are available at soundstrue.com/vibration-of-grace-bonus.

Taking Yourself Out of a Harm-Filled Moment

As you deepen your soul retrieval practice, you will find that your relationship with your younger self will grow stronger. Sometimes there is an immediate bond, and other times it takes a few sessions of practice before your younger self will step forward completely. Remember that you are in a trust-building process, and this requires patience. I promise you the child inside wants to feel loved, seen, cared for. If you keep to your practice, trust will happen. Once this is achieved and they come to you readily, you will be able to return to a moment of harm and disrupt the memory to free yourself.

Here are two stories of this next level of soul retrieval practice, one from someone I have guided and one share from my own life.

My client spent his babyhood and toddler years with a mother who was addicted to heroin. He had many painful memories, and one in particular that he was fixated upon. Often his mind would travel back to a memory of his toddler self being trapped in a high chair for hours and hours, crying to his mother, who was in a heroin-induced stupor, laid out on a couch in front of his chair. His father, who did not live with them, came to see what was happening after trying to call repeatedly and getting no answer. He found his young son in an inconsolable state, wearing a diaper past full, thirsty, hungry, and afraid. He took his son out of the chair and took him away from his mother. My client never lived with his mother again.

There are many wounds here, being a small child trapped in a high chair is one, and it is the place he would return to often, with feelings of despair and bouts of suicidal ideation. After a few sessions working together, he felt he was ready to return to that moment to retrieve his toddler self. We began our session with deep breathing and affirmation, noticing the body, bringing breath to each noticing. Then I invited him to remember and imagine.

Together, we entered the room where his toddler self was waiting to be rescued. I instructed him to free the child, to take him into his arms and leave the house. I asked him to place the child on the grass out front and then to return to the house to grab the high chair and bring it outside. I told him I would care for the baby and he should take the high chair a safe distance away and break it into tiny pieces by smashing it against the ground. Then I told him to pick up his baby self and take him to a park nearby to rest and play. He asked about his mother passed out on the couch, and I reminded him that this was about centering and rescuing his little boy self, that he was the only one we could save. We did this work together in guided meditation, with visioning and imagination.

Afterward, I slowly brought him back to the present moment. He left my studio with instructions: have a good meal, hydrate well, and spend the rest of the day choosing easy activities. I checked in with him a few days later to ask him about the memory. He shared that it had left him completely, that he was free of that chair because that chair no longer existed. In the time since we did this ritual together, he has practiced it on his own and freed more parts of himself. He no longer has suicidal ideation, and he is giving himself the daily joy and practice of a loving relationship and children of his own. He still grieves sometimes for his mom, but that grief no longer drives his behavior.

From my personal journey, I am about to tell a story about child sexual abuse. Please take care of yourself and listen to your body. Stop reading if your body says stop. You can skip over this story or return to it later if you wish.

There was a time in my life when I did not own my body. Pleasure was difficult for me, sometimes not possible. I trusted few people, and I struggled with relationships. The memories of being sexually abused were all-consuming; I could not escape it. My five-year-old self was suffering from being terrorized daily by an older cousin. My eleven-year-old self was grappling with a dim memory of my father on top of her, knowing trespass had happened but not being able to recall.

I decided to begin with the clearest memory, inviting the voice of my five-year-old self into the room. I followed the instructions from Grace that I have shared with you and began my soul retrieval work. I created a safe place for my five-year-old self to tell me what was wrong. It was painful and profoundly difficult. I cried and stayed with her. After a few weeks of practice, she would come to me readily to be comforted. I imagined holding her close, kissing her face, and singing her to sleep. When I was ready, I returned to the place and time of my cousin assaulting me, and I rescued little gina.

I did this ritual while resting in my bed, where I felt comfortable and safe. I set my timer for thirty minutes. I began to imagine returning as my grown self to the room where I was repeatedly molested. I opened the door and pushed the one hurting me out of the room. I did not look at his face. I picked up my baby girl self, and I imagined the weight of her body, her arms wrapping around my neck, her legs wrapping around my waist, as we left that room, never to return. I kept my focus on her and gave no more attention to the person who hurt her. I imagined taking her to a bath full of bubbles, and after receiving her permission, I washed her body with great care. When the timer chimed, I thanked her for being so brave and told her that it was my honor to care for her. I told her she would never be harmed again.

I created loving boundaries where she got to play and rest and just be five. After a few weeks of this practice, my fear and avoidance of sexual pleasure dissipated. After a few months, I felt my body become mine again. Thoughts of pleasure and acts of desire were free from fear and terrifying imagery. My five-year-old self was finally home, safe with me.

Integration

The ritual of soul retrieval will sometimes yield quick results, and you will begin to feel a sense of relief almost immediately. And there may be times when you must go back to a hard place to get yourself. This is part of the process of integration. I can go years without needing to engage in a soul retrieval ritual, and then some painful happening will send my baby girl self back to her post on the doorstep, waiting for her mother's return. When this happens, I go and get her, as she responds now to the sound of my voice. I know what to say to assure her that she is cherished and that I need her with me. Keep speaking love to your younger selves. Tell them that they deserve every good thing. This helps them feel safe and seen and gives them permission to stay present with you.

5

Sound and Repair:
The Vibrational Power
of True Apology

I n October 2018, I went to Kigali, Rwanda, to meet with Rev. Philbert Kalisa, founder and director of REACH Rwanda, an organization formed after the Rwandan genocide and dedicated to the ongoing work of healing and reconciliation. In Rwanda, the language of "perpetrator" and "victim" is used to describe the Hutu tribe militia and deputized Hutu (perpetrators) who murdered over 800,000 people from the Tutsi tribe (victims) over the course of three months in 1994, during the Rwandan civil war. There is a much longer, complex story here, rooted in colonialism, economic disparity, and fearmongering. I am sharing a broad view for context. In the years since the Rwandan genocide, there has been a profound effort for peace, healing, and reconciliation in Rwanda for the Rwandan people and a dedicated interest in letting the world community know what happened there so it never happens again. I had read that the children from the Hutu tribe were marrying the children from the Tutsi tribe, going into business together, sharing resources, trying to live and love beyond the unimaginable horror of genocide. I wanted to experience and witness the amazing work that created the conditions for this healing. My intention was to learn all I could and bring that learning back home to the United States to prayerfully be in service to the profound healing that needs to happen in my country.

When I arrived in Rwanda, I was immediately taken to the Kigali Genocide Memorial, where the remains of over 250,000 people are interred. The last room of the memorial museum is dedicated to the children who were killed. I was half aware that I was lying on the floor of that room, wailing. I had a similar reaction at the National Memorial for Peace and Justice, in Montgomery, Alabama. I was overcome by the inhumanity and senselessness. Wailing was the proper response. After a while, still laid out on the floor in the children's memorial room, I heard Grace telling me to listen. As I quieted, I could hear a buzzing sound with a high pitch, almost like singing. It calmed my spirit and helped me witness those who had died. I said prayers, touched the ground, and gave thanks to the ancestors of that land for allowing me to be there.

The next day Rev. Kalisa invited me to join a storytelling circle at REACH, for people who had survived the genocidal war. There would be an interpreter in the room so that I could listen and share. There were about fifty people present; some were Hutus and Tutsis directly connected by violence. There was a man and a woman sitting to my left laughing and talking in Kinyarwanda. The love between them was palpable. The woman had scars on her face and an indentation in her skull. Rev. Kalisa shared with me that the wounds on the woman's face were caused by a machete and that her friend sitting next to her was the one who inflicted those wounds and left her for dead. This information left me speechless and confused. I could feel their friendship and affection for each other. How was this possible? We opened the circle with a grounding meditation, shared with me through an interpreter, and we began our introductions.

The two friends were asked if they would tell me their story. They said yes enthusiastically and asked if I would let people in the United States know about their journey. I thanked them and told them I would be honored to share every word. They began by telling me that they were neighbors in 1994, before violence erupted around them one April morning. She was thirteen and he was eighteen, and they saw each other every day, mostly in passing. She was in school, and he was contemplating joining the army, hoping to bring some structure to his life. They were not politicized and dimly aware of tribal tensions. She was Tutsi, and he was Hutu. They lived in a rural area outside of Kigali.

The day that violence spread through Rwanda like a brush fire, she remembers waking to screams and witnessing neighbors turn against each other. She lost all her family that day and was trying to escape her village when she came upon her Hutu neighbor, wielding a machete and swinging it on anyone he recognized as Tutsi. This was when he shared that he was told he and his family would be killed if he did not obey the orders of the Hutu militia. He went on to say that he lost himself that day and in the days to follow. He joined the mob fueled by hatred and bloodlust and felt completely separated from his sense of reason and morality. He saw her and used his machete on her body. She fell to the ground, and he kept moving. She survived by pretending to be dead.

She sheltered in a storeroom that was owned by a Hutu neighbor who risked their life to save hers and a few others. He fled Rwanda for Uganda when the Rwandan Patriotic Front ended the genocide by defeating the civilian and military authorities responsible for the killing campaign. He returned to Rwanda a year later, confessed his crimes, and spent some years in prison. While in prison, he thought of her often. When released, he returned to his village and learned that she had survived. He asked for permission to see her, and she declined. He shared that daily he would stand outside of the fence that circled her home with his hands in prayer position, head bowed, asking her permission to speak with her. She looked at me and with an interpreter's help told me there was no way she was going to speak with him. She would close her curtains every time he came by, hoping he would leave her alone. She then said it was God who changed her mind. She prayed and received inner guidance to allow him to enter her home. He apologized to her for his heinous behavior and asked her what he could do to make amends. She felt his sincerity and believed his words, and she did not know how to move forward. Together they began to attend meetings at REACH Rwanda and learned new practices of storytelling, listening, and accountability. He told us that now he and his wife visit with her often, bringing her food, medicine, whatever she needs. They have become family.

After they shared their testimony, Rev. Kalisa asked me if I would offer a sound-healing practice. I invited them to sit side by side in the center and the group to gather around them. With their permission, I laid hands, one on the shoulder of each, and began to sound and tone, guided by Grace. I invited the group into a soft and constant hum, as I stood behind her first and toned into the back of her skull and neck and then did the same for him. I began to sound into the wounds on her face, as I rested my hand on his shoulder. I will never forget the pure feeling of peace between them. There was no presence of rancor or fear, only love.

I left Rwanda with a renewed knowing around what is possible, having witnessed people who are healing from the unimaginable. While there, I heard many stories of intentional repair, of people desiring the freedom that only healing can bring. True apology carries a vibration that creates a divine point of entry for connection, and it is the beginning place that makes repair and a forgiveness practice possible.

Accountability Is a Healer

I want to tell you about my personal experience with true apology, and how my mother and I found our way back to each other. When I was 43 years old, I told my mother she was the first person to break my heart. I told her I had been on a healing journey since I was six years old, the day she left, when I heard Grace speak for the first time. She listened quietly and with complete attention as I told her about all that had happened to me because of her leaving us. I told her about being sexually abused, about the constant narratives of feeling unworthy, unlovable, too big, too much, and not enough. She listened and witnessed my grief, anger, and practice. My mother waited until I finished speaking. She took a deep breath and spoke love into the room: "I am so sorry for hurting you. I am sorry I abandoned you and caused so much pain. Please forgive me. How do we heal our relationship?"

My mother did not make excuses or defend her choices. She held space with me and listened. She did not shift focus to her own stories. She stayed present and curious about what I had to say. My mother's apology resonated deep inside my being, and we began a new relationship that day, anchored in accountability and a desire to repair what was broken between us. We started to meet regularly for conversations about generational grief. We prayed and visioned a new legacy of love and care for my daughter and all my mother's grandchildren. Over time, I was able to receive my mother's stories of her own journey through grief and despair. This allowed me to think of her as separate from me, as someone more than the one who birthed me and harmed me. Seeing my mom as a separate being with her own troubles and interior life helped me to individuate and to become more myself. I began to understand more fully that I was in control of my choices and that I was free to have a different response to my mother, one not rooted in anger. I was 49 when my mother died. We were still in our practice of loving repair. Our accountability ritual allowed my mama to release much of the shame she carried for leaving her children, and it allowed me to properly grieve her passing without old resentment blocking my release.

I miss my mother every single day. The work we did together allowed us to reclaim our relationship. And sometimes I still have to go and rescue my baby girl self from a choice she made, because healing takes time. We broke a painful cycle for generations to come, and that is everything.

We use the language of "true apology," as sometimes apologies are devoid of feelings of contrition, and therefore not real. I used to be terrible at apologizing. When someone would tell me something I did or said caused them harm, I would say things like, "That's your shit, not mine," or "There are two sides to every story," and my personal favorite, "I'm sorry if you think I hurt you." I was dismissive, self-righteous, and terrified of being seen as wrong. I could hear Grace telling me to slow down and listen; my fear created enough noise to drown out this wisdom. The accountability practice with my mother and the love of good friends calling me in and not shaming me helped me to learn how to hear and then respond when I cause harm. My love for my daughter taught me how to apologize well. Parenting is absolutely the hardest job I have ever had, and sometimes I make mistakes. I will apologize to my child when I say or do things that are not in alignment with love. This, as I have shared, is very different from the parenting I received. Another painful cycle broken.

———————— Ritual ————————

TO ACCESS THE POWER OF APOLOGY

I've had many clients over the years express their inability to apologize and a desire to learn how to be in right relationship when they cause harm. Here are some practices we call *Apology Alchemy rituals*: one practice will guide you through giving an apology, and another will teach you how to care for yourself when you want an apology that you will not be receiving. Please be gentle with yourself and curious about what may be revealed as you allow us to guide you.

Tools

- a journal or recording device
- a timer with a soft ring
- a handheld mirror or bathroom vanity mirror

Eventually, you may do this work with a friend, sibling, or partner. That person will be your mirror, and you will be theirs. To begin, however, I encourage you to make this a solo practice.

Preparation

Before you face the mirror, find your way to a comfortable position, sitting or lying down. Leaning into your conscious breath practice, inhale deeply now through your nose and exhale through your mouth. Taking your time, please cycle this breath practice and notice how you are feeling at this moment. Breathe and consider. Notice your body, and notice your mind. Bring your full awareness to breathing, inhaling deeply through your nose and exhaling slowly through your mouth. Please repeat this pattern at your own pace.

Then open your journal and record your answers to these questions:

- What happens in your body when you think about apologizing?

- Was apology part of the rules of engagement in your home growing up?

- Did your primary caregivers ever apologize?

- Can you think of someone you feel owes you an apology?

Please breathe deeply and notice how and what you are feeling. Try to allow any feelings connected to memories to pass through; try not to stay with one story. If this proves difficult, turn your full attention to your breath, as you inhale deeply through your nose and exhale slowly through your mouth. Breathe and notice. Stay with your breath, and notice your shoulders, the back of your neck, your stomach area. Are you holding any tension in these areas? Now, your lower back, legs, down to the soles of your feet—take in your body and continue to inhale deeply through your nose and to exhale through your mouth. Tension can show up in the body as tight muscles, light-headedness, nausea, deep fatigue. Your intentional breathing practice should help settle these feelings if they arise.

Listen. Grace wants to talk about shame. I always thought of shame as something to be dispatched quickly and cleanly from the body, mind, and spirit of whoever came to me for healing work. The pervasive and insatiable presence of shame, like a blight that creates psychogenic pain and inflammation in the body, served no purpose and needed to be gone. A beloved told me recently that shame is a social emotion that does have a purpose. In its proper place, shame helps us to be aware of our inter-dependence. It can support mindful behavior and keep us from acting exclusively from our own self-interest. And shame has been co-opted, used as a weapon to control, manipulate, and cause harm. If we act outside of our integrity, we may feel shame about that. But shame does not have to mean that we go into a spiral of self-loathing or that someone will put us on blast via social media or gossiping. Shame is a primary reason why people have difficulty apologizing. When we hear we have caused harm, whatever shame we may walk with becomes activated and can take over the moment. We lose our sense of self, afraid to be seen as less than who we wish to be, afraid our actions mean we don't get to be loved and belong.

We can absolutely learn how to keep shame out of our body and center love in our exchanges, even the painful and difficult ones.

Ritual

Keep your journal or recording device close. Lift your mirror and begin to gaze at your reflection. (If it is more comfortable for you to use a mirror attached to a wall, please do.) Look at your face, your eyes, nose, mouth, forehead, chin, ears, the base of your throat. You may also touch your face, move the tips of your fingers over your face and feel your skin. As you look and touch, practice conscious breathing, inhaling through your nose and exhaling audibly through your mouth. Set your intention: You are going to practice apologizing. You are going to notice any resistance to this practice and where this resistance comes from. Make the agreement with yourself that you will take care of your body and that there is no rush nor pressure involved with this ritual. When you are ready, move to the next step.

Remember a moment of conflict—someone who may have wanted or asked you for an apology—and go with your first memory, what the body reveals. Whether you apologized or not, you are going to practice apologizing now. Trust your body wisdom; the memory that rises is your point of entry.

Set your timer for five minutes, and make sure the ring is on low volume and pleasant to hear.

Gazing into your eyes, say this sentence out loud, which begins with the person's name:

_____ , *I'm sorry I hurt you. I'm sorry that I caused you harm.*

Repeat this sentence, pause, breathe, and repeat again. When the timer chimes, write in your journal any feelings, thoughts, or memories that came to mind as you engaged this practice. Notice grief, anger, ambivalence, any feelings that rise, and record them in your journal.

When ready, set your timer for five minutes, and look into the mirror again. Inhale deeply through your nose and exhale slowly through your mouth. Say the same person's name and repeat this sentence out loud:

_____ , *I'm sorry that I hurt you. I take full responsibility for my choices. I am not ashamed or afraid to apologize. How may I make amends?*

Stay with your breath practice and pause as needed. Remember: there is no rush and no pressure here. When the timer chimes, return to your journal and record what you wish to remember. Return to conscious breathing and take a few minutes to listen and be with your body.

When you are ready, set your timer for five minutes, and turn toward your mirror to look into your eyes, saying your full name, while you repeat this sentence out loud:

_____ , *I am so sorry that I hurt you. I love you, I care for you, and I will protect you from harm from now on.*

Breathe, pause, and repeat this sentence to yourself, gazing into your eyes. Practice not judging the feelings that surface in your body during this ritual. When the timer chimes, write down your experience with this ritual, any counter narratives that may have surfaced, and your body's response to your words.

Closing

After you journal, close the ritual by thanking yourself out loud for your courage, curiosity, and commitment to hold yourself in love. Go gently and generously into your day, pledging that you will take good and deep care of yourself.

Healing Without Receiving a True Apology

The energy of harm can tether us to each other; apology supports the unbraiding of this energy. Often it is not possible to receive an apology from someone who has harmed us, sometimes because the person isn't capable and sometimes because the person dies or leaves our life.

In one such example, I will share a story of a client who was unconsciously longing for an apology from her mother because of something that happened when she was a teenager. We began working together shortly after her 55th birthday; her mother had passed away some years before. My client came to me seeking to understand why she was not able to allow herself to be in a romantic relationship. She kept finding herself attracted to people who ultimately decided they wanted friendship only. After a few sessions of talk therapy, she was surprised to discover that she had resistance to being in a relationship. She came to me for a sound-healing session, hoping to discover the reason why.

Grace guided us to her teenage years, to a crush she had then on one of her teachers in high school. She wrote in her journal that she was in love with this woman and that she wanted to kiss her. She would volunteer to stay after class to straighten up at the end of each day just so she could spend time in her teacher's presence. She shared with me that she thought her teacher was completely unaware of her feelings and that the energy between them was always appropriate. She became a model student and was always the first one to raise her hand in class and to volunteer for any afterschool happenings. Once, her teacher called her home to speak with her about a class trip, and her mother answered the phone. She came to the phone blushing, clearly excited and eager to take the call, and her mother recognized the energy. The next day her mother revealed that she had read her journal while she was at school. She was devastated by her mother's trespass of her privacy and deeply ashamed by what her mother had read. She was unable to respond when her mother told her she would not tolerate *that* kind of behavior in her house, that it was a sin and she never wanted to hear about it again.

When she first came to work with me, my client had a dim memory of this exchange. She did not realize until now the impact her mother's words had on her spirit. She said her mother never raised her voice, and so it did not feel like she was being harmed. With this memory came an old sense of self-loathing that she was not aware of. She realized her mother's response created a feeling of internalized homophobia in her psyche. I helped her to realize she had made an unconscious pact with loneliness the day her mother read her journal and discovered her secret. It was one way to deal with the shame of her mother's disapproval and to ensure she would still receive her mother's love.

My client began dating women after graduating from college and had had a few girlfriends. She was unconsciously bound by her mother's desire for silence and never found the courage to tell her the truth about her life. She did not realize, at the time, how much she wanted her mother's approval.

Big or Little Grief

Over time, through soul retrieval rituals and wailing, my client discovered that when working with the body there is no such thing as big or little grief. Most of us have been weaned on binary thinking, which can cause us to measure everything. We measure painful happenings and decide what is relevant and deserves our attention by how "big" or "little" the moment of impact. My client had minimized what happened with her mother, and it was that moment of harm that shaped her entire relationship to romance and pleasure. Once she realized how much her mother's actions had hurt her, she wanted an apology. But because her mother was no longer living, my client had to heal the space between them on her own and bring herself to a place of self-acceptance and love without the sound of her mother's voice giving her permission. I am privileged to share that after months of consistent practice she was able to allow the love she so desired to come into her life, and she has a daily practice around blessing the space between herself and her mother.

Measuring Harm

Dear family, please pause here for a moment and bring awareness to your breath. Inhale deeply through your nose and exhale slowly through your mouth; cycle this breath. We want to underscore how my client did not comprehend the degree of harm her mother's words caused because her mother did not raise her voice. Some harm happens quietly, and because it does not announce itself like cymbals crashing, we miss it. Although our mind does not grasp the happening, our body absorbs the destructive energy. Our rituals of care help us to be in a deeper relationship with our body, which sharpens our awareness so that we are better able to feel and name harm as it is happening.

———— Ritual ————
FOR BLESSING THE SPACE BETWEEN

The ritual of blessing the space between us and someone who has died or is incapable of owning their behavior and apologizing is not about the other person. This is an important knowing, dear family: you are the one you are liberating here, not the person who harmed you. You center yourself and your care by staying with your own story. When working with harm caused by loved ones who have died, you may feel that you are dishonoring their memory in some way. It can feel easier to ignore your needs by saying to yourself that they did the best they could. This is probably true, yet this truth will not necessarily heal the wound caused by their actions.

By centering yourself you will not be distracted by feelings you may have for the person in question. Do not imagine or lean into their story. Stay with the one inside you who is still holding what happened, and practice this ritual.

Tools

- a journal

Preparation

Turn your attention to your thoughts, and notice when memories of unresolved conflict come to mind. Sometimes harm can feel quite present in your mind, and sometimes you don't notice how much a thought has become part of the fabric of your interior life, a seemingly innocuous narrative pilfering energy daily and dictating your responses. Maybe you shrug off the experience as something you just have to get over, since the person involved is not available to you. Practice noticing if these thoughts come to your mind as you move through everyday things, like grocery shopping, getting yourself or your children ready for the day, watching television. Repetitive thoughts can be your body's way of communicating to you that you need care around what happened.

When you are able to identify the person and the moment, write these thoughts and memories in your journal. Do not think of the totality of your relationship with this person; isolate the moment of harm. In the case of my client and her mother's destructive language, there were many moments of love and care. The harm was not the all of their journey, and it still needed to be circled and deactivated so that she could be free of her mother's opinion and choose her own walk.

After recording your memory in your journal, turn to a new page and write three sentences that elicit a feeling of peace and finality in your body. These can be sentences you create or lines from your favorite poems, quotes, lyrics, things your grandmother or beloved teachers told you. Here are some examples from my practice:

- *I bless the space between us; may we both be circled in light.*
- *Mercy lives in the space between us; I release all harm to Grace.*
- *There is only peace between us; I release you to your journey.*

Ritual

When the unhealed moment rises in your mind, say one of your prepared sentences out loud, and marry this sentence with a gesture, such as fingers touching the base of your throat or a hand over your beating heart or solar plexus. Practice speaking aloud while engaging this gesture. After a while, the gesture will be enough to shift your thoughts toward what you wish to think about as the memory of harm begins to fade.

Closing

The ritual of blessing can be an ongoing offering; lean into it as you need. You will look up one day and notice you have not thought about the harmful thing that happened in a good long while.

My Story of Healing Without a True Apology

The story I will share from my life is about sexual abuse and incest. Please take care of yourself, family. You can always skip or come back to this section. Check in with your body and notice how you are feeling before you continue. Please trust your body wisdom.

In my healing practice, sexual abuse, assault, rape, incest, and child molestation are most often the trauma that brings people to my table. Inside the rituals we offer is a pathway to reclaiming and owning your body and disrupting the trauma. I experience this freedom in my own body, and I have participated in helping to liberate others of the festering wounds from sexual assault. I have been doing my own work to heal from sexual abuse for many years.

I have shared my stories often, in circle work and on stages during my concerts, and as I prepare to write my story down for the first time, I am noticing a desire to protect my father's memory. I do not want people to read this and think horrible things about him, because I love him dearly. Still, I know that my stories of healing are of service and must be shared. Both things are true.

My father died when I was twelve years old. When I was in my early thirties, I began to have memories about him that frightened and confused me. I thought I was losing my sanity. This thought was easier to embrace than the memories that began to flood my mind whenever I thought of him—which was daily because his picture was centered in a place of honor on my ancestor altar. When I looked at my father's picture, I would be bombarded by images of his hands touching a vagina clearly belonging to a little girl. I knew these images were of things that happened to me, and I did not know how to face it.

I asked Grace, Why now? Why were these memories coming for me now? Grace replied, *Mercy.* She told me that mercy is a being that protects us from bodily memory our minds were not able to hold and that if my body and mind were revealing something, I was going to be able to look at what had happened between me and my father and rescue my child self.

Alongside the images of his hands in my vagina, there was a memory I could never fully access. I was eleven years old and in bed with him. He was naked under his robe. I remember hating this robe that never stayed tied, always flying open and revealing his penis. He was on top of me. I remember that I had clothes on and that he kept licking his lips and kissing my face. It was a game that felt terrible in my body, yet I stayed and giggled and pretended with him that the game was a good one. So complex. The multitude of feelings: fear, grief, shame, and the desire to be seen and loved by him. At the time, I did not have language for all these feelings that were braided together by my adoration and love. The memory goes dark after the kissing game, and I am still not able to recall what happened next. I am grateful to mercy. Clearly, I can be free without knowing all of the details. We do not have to remember the abuse that happened to us to release it and banish it from the body.

I began soul retrieval rituals to return to the abuse with my father, and I took my baby-girl selves out of those moments. I returned more than once to get my eleven-year-old self from my father's bed and take her to places of safety and care. I also did the ritual I shared with you to move anger. I broke so many plates, smashing them to pieces as I allowed myself to get angry at my father. I took his picture from my ancestor altar and put it away where I would not have to see his face. Alongside my sound-healing rituals, I received acupuncture from a masterful practitioner and found a somatic therapist who could hold space with me. Over time, the memories of abuse began to fade, and then left me completely.

The years of working my healing practice have gifted me with ease and full access to my expressions of desire and pleasure. I have full sovereignty over my body now. My father's picture is back on my ancestor altar, and I have no feelings of anger toward him. The rituals of loving myself forward created the opportunity to feel compassion for him. I did not rush to this place. I allowed myself the time I needed. I did not force-feed a forgiveness practice on my baby girl selves. I practiced moving the anger, and I allowed my grief to have full reign until it passed.

During my rituals, I desired my father's witnessing and apology, so I blessed the space between us throughout the day. I began to imagine conversations we would have if he were still alive. My father was more than an abuser; who would he be now if he had lived past 49? I began to vision him years in the future, how he may have grown past depression and addiction to a place of understanding and self-forgiveness. It was *this* man I imagine moving into his own healing journey. It is this version of my father I imagine him loving his grandchildren and great grandchildren—proud, happy, and released from turmoil. This is the man who occupies space on my altar and in my heart. My father healed, whole, liberated, and free. I hold him in this space with the power of my word, imagination, and conjure.

And so, I am a living testimony of the power of this work we offer to you. When I began to practice, I had days where I thought I would never be free of the harm my father caused. Dear family, the memories that used to haunt me no longer have power. I actually never think about what happened between my father and me unless I am sharing the story. You can also be free of the terrible things that happened to you. I promise.

part three

SOUNDING

—— *into the* ——

BODY

somebody told me that the darkest hour comes right before the dawn
and I would find my way back to myself if I could just hold on,
hold on, hold on, til the light—
and it's gonna be alright, cause love is on your side,
don't fear your life, it's gonna be alright

6

Sound and Vital Organs: The Universe Inside You

Beloved family, as we shared in this book's introduction, we are currently in deep practice to create rituals anchored in vibration, touch, and other languages that can be sourced for healing. The following rituals are centered on the sound of the voice. Please skip this chapter if this will not serve you.

When we go to speak, our breath vibrates our vocal cords (the small bands of muscle inside the larynx) and engages the vocal resonator system (the nose, throat, and mouth) to produce sound that is unique and cannot be replicated. There are physical reasons why the voice is like a sonic fingerprint—the shape of the mouth, neck, vocal tract, and chest, the positioning of the tongue, bone structure, bone density, muscle tension—all these things affect pitch, timbre, and tone of the voice. When we turn our full attention to the human voice, we hear layers of sound. Words are vital, certainly, and the sound inside the word is how we know when truth is being spoken, by the way it lands in our body and makes us feel. There are energetic and spiritual reasons why your voice belongs to you as well. All our life experiences inform our sound. The depth and breadth of your journey is inside the sound of you.

Consider How You Feel About Your Voice

Take a moment now to consider the following. How do you feel about your voice? What is your relationship to the sound that carries the words you choose? Think of times when you are most comfortable bringing your voice into a room and times when you don't feel safe or find it difficult to speak. Please write your answers to these questions in your journal.

Grace tells me that our relationship to our voice begins with the first cry. Did someone pick us up, hold us close, and tend to our needs? Was our cry answered? As we grew, were we listened to, encouraged to share and tell? Did our no or yes matter? Were we told to shut up, be quiet, be seen but not heard? Or greeted with curiosity and "say more about that"? All these possibilities create our connection to our sound and how we use and don't use the power of our voice.

As you recall the happenings that shaped your feelings about your voice, try not to get caught in memory. The story, your story, is profoundly important and has a place. For our work, we want to bring this information about how your relationship to your voice was shaped without getting caught in any stories of harm. If you have difficulty with this invitation to stay in the present moment as you are looking to the past, please pause and turn your attention to this conscious breath practice to gather yourself.

Inhale deeply through your nose and exhale slowly through your mouth. Cycle this breath five times. Consider your body and the space you occupy. Orient yourself by noticing light, colors, temperature; take in your surroundings. When you are ready, return to the ritual.

Our sound is a gift. The evidence of this is everywhere present. If we can be fooled into thinking our voice does not matter, we will not speak against injustice. We will not cast, conjure, or declare our right to love and be loved where we stand, how we choose, and in all the ways we need to thrive. Let the sound guide us to the word and the word guide us on the path, as we learn to speak our deliverance from oppression and tyranny using our sound in service to love whenever and wherever we can.

——————— Ritual ———————

FOR SOUNDING INTO YOUR BODY

Dear family, in this ritual you will be sounding into the five organs considered vital for life—the liver, heart, lungs, brain, kidneys—and your perineum and pancreas. You will be working with vowels, humming, and visioning. There are thousands of vowels in the languages of the world; for this offering, we will work with the basic vowels for written English: A, E, I, O, U. We work with vowels because of how the sound is produced: the sound is made without closing the mouth or any part of the throat, which creates an opportunity for the uninterrupted flow of energy. Vowels are embedded in our consciousness and generally easy to access. Grace says that vowel sounds have summoning power we will use to call out energy that does not belong. Our organs can house energy that depletes our vitality. This ritual gives voice to this energy so that it can be released, and then we can begin new practices of restoration anchored in awareness.

Humming is something my grandmother did to calm her nerves and center her spirit. Humming is now recognized as having a direct and healing effect on the vagus nerve, the main nerve of the parasympathetic nervous system. The vagus nerve begins at the base of the brain and passes through the neck, chest, stomach, and colon, and connects to the heart, lungs, and kidneys. The vagal nerves regulate internal organ functions, digestion, heart rate, respiratory rate, as well as certain reflex actions, coughing, sneezing, and swallowing. A regular practice of sounding and humming into our internal organs will support a healthy vagal tone.

As porous, interconnected beings, many of us are carrying more stress than we realize. It is a heightened time of fear in the world for myriad reasons, and even those of us who consider ourselves relatively healthy are breathing the same air, thick with grief and attrition. Even if you never read, watch, or listen to the news, you still feel the daily happenings. We are expending much energy navigating all manner of instability. Taking time to massage our organs with sound will restore and replenish our internal energy reserves.

Harmonizing the Cells

With this ritual you will place intentional sound into your cells. When you commit to regular practice, you can bring your body into a kind of tonal alignment, where the individual sounds and frequencies of your organs, blood flow, chakras, and narratives move in glorious rhythm together, a spiritual symmetry of harmonious sound that one can feel when you enter a room.

As I write, I am seeing an image of visible sound waves, rolling for miles and miles, touching skin, hearts, minds, lifting spirits, inspiring folks to join the *heaven is this moment* chorus of voices, and every other word sung or spoken is peace, power, and healing grace for all. Let's begin.

Tools

- a journal and pen
- a nourishing meal
- water for drinking
- a medicine bath of one cup of sea salt and one cup of baking soda

Preparation

Read through the ritual a few times and practice the vowels. Locate the organs you will be sounding into and learn more about how these organs work together to serve your body by doing some research.

You will need private space, a comfortable place to rest, as you move through your ritual. Have a nourishing meal prepared for after you close, and take time to reflect and record what you may learn, discover, release, and receive. Try to do the ritual from beginning to close, but do not worry if you must work in segments. The entire practice may be ninety minutes or more. Plan to take a medicine bath or rinse after you close (using one cup of sea salt and one cup of baking soda). If you choose to rinse, you may fill a big pot with warm water, stir your ingredients in the pot until they dissolve, take this into the shower and gather handfuls of the mixture to pour over the back of your neck, throat, shoulders, and full body. If you choose a bath, pour the ingredients into a full tub of water and rest as long as you wish.

Ritual

Open this ritual by giving thanks to the ancestors of the land that is supporting your life and practice. Then, honor your ancestors, those who have come before you, and those who may follow after. Set your intention for this ritual: to sound into your body and vision your vital organs, perineum, and pancreas vibrantly healthy and at ease. Then, sitting comfortably or lying down, bring your conscious breathing practice forward. Inhale deeply through your nose and exhale slowly through your mouth; cycle this breath five times. Soften or close your eyes. Relax your jaw by creating space between your tongue and the roof of your mouth. Breathe.

Slowly begin to guide your mind around your body. Begin at the pelvic floor and travel up the front of your body, past the navel, stomach, center of your chest, the base of your throat, your chin, between your eyes, forehead, to the crown of your head. Then travel down your back body. Pause and breathe deeply into your shoulders. Then follow your spine, vertebrae by vertebrae, to the tip of your sacrum. When you feel relaxed and ready, bring your awareness to your perineum, the space between the anus and genitals. Breathe and consider your perineum. From the perineum, guide your mind toward your liver, located on the right side of your body, just under your ribs. Breathe and consider your liver. Then move to the left side of your body and locate your beating heart. Rest your hand or your mind there while you breathe and consider your heart. Guide your mind now to your lungs, which live on either side of the breastbone in your chest. Take your time and stay with your conscious breathing as you consider your lungs. After your lungs, bring your awareness to your brain, specifically, the pineal gland, which rests deep in the center of the brain. Imagine a pyramid shape inside, where the top of the triangle begins at the center of your eyes connecting above the ear on either side of your skull and the pineal gland lives at the center of the pyramid. Breathe and consider your pineal gland. Then bring your awareness to your kidneys, located near your back body on either side of your spine, below your rib cage, and behind your belly. Breathe and consider your kidneys. Now, find your way to your pancreas, which touches the left and right side of the body, just behind your stomach, close to your liver. Breathe deeply and consider your pancreas. As you move deeper into this ritual, please adapt this practice to support what works for your body.

Bring the vowels A, E, I, O, U to your mind; say them out loud and repeat. Now sing each vowel on the exhale. Any note that is comfortable is fine, and you may use the same note for each vowel.

> Inhale deeply; exhale a long AAAAAAAAAAA
> Inhale deeply; exhale a long EEEEEEEEEEEEE
> Inhale deeply; exhale a long IIIIIIIIIIIIIIIIIIIIIIII
> Inhale deeply; exhale a long OOOOOOOOOOO
> Inhale deeply; exhale a long UUUUUUUUUUU

The Liver and the Vowel A. The liver filters the blood in the body and breaks down chemical substances like alcohol and prescription drugs. The liver produces a fluid called bile, necessary for the digestive process. I hear often from practitioners of traditional medicines that the liver also filters and will house our anger. Grace agrees with this assessment and reminds us that the liver is also known as the most "forgiving" organ, as a healthy liver can regenerate itself from a third of the original mass.

Let us sound into your liver. When you are ready, rest your hand over your liver (just above your stomach, under your right rib cage); if you are not able to lay hands, then your attention and intention will do just fine. Close or soften your eyes and begin to guide your mind to your liver and breathe deeply. Imagine your dark, healthy liver, and imagine you feel your liver under your palm as you breathe and listen. Begin your long exhalation of the vowel A, inhaling deeply and exhaling AAAAAAAAAAAA, and repeat, AAAAAAAAAAAA with full focus on your liver. You are sounding A into this organ. Exhale, AAAAAAAAAAA three times, and then pause, listen, and breathe. Be curious. Do not decide what, if anything, should be revealed. Practice being a witness to yourself. Notice any stories, words, songs that may rise to your mind. Just notice and stay with your breath.

Now, repeat the long exhaling of A into your liver, and this time, imagine you can see the sound of your voice entering your liver. See the voice as streams of your favorite color, like the sun's rays coming through a window at dawn. See these colors of your sound moving into your liver. Imagine that this beauty will dispel any memory, story, word, or energy that does not feel good, loving, joyous. Cycle this vision, animated by your voice, through your liver, exhaling a long AAAAAAAAAA, on repeat, five times. See the colors from your sounding of the vowel A filling your liver to overflow with energy moving like waves, undulating over and over. When you finish your fifth sounding of the vowel A, pause, rest, and breathe. Check in with yourself. Make sure you are still in the most comfortable position. Have some water, and then continue.

The Kidneys and the Vowel E. The kidneys cleanse the blood of toxins and transform waste into urine. In 24 hours, the kidneys filter close to 150 quarts of blood; one or two quarts will become urine. We have discovered that the energy of prolonged shame in the body will collect in the kidneys and cause harm there. Let us sound into your kidneys. Bring your awareness to your back body, locating your kidneys alongside your spine, just below your ribs. If you are comfortably able, place your hands over your kidneys. You may need to sit forward to do this. If not, no worries; simply hold your kidneys in your mind. From inside of your conscious breathing practice, inhale deeply and then exhale a long EEEEEEEEE, with full focus on your kidneys. Exhale the vowel E three times. Then pause, listen, breathe. Be curious and allow your response. Notice thoughts and feelings; be with your body and witness.

You are going to sound E into your kidneys again, and as you did with the vowel A and your liver, you are going to imagine the sound of your voice entering your kidneys as streams of color and light. Use this image and sound to move any energy in your kidneys that needs to move. Inhale deeply, and exhale EEEEEEEEEE into your kidneys five times, seeing the light-filled sound of the vowel E move across and through your kidneys, back and forth, energy leaving and then replenished from the inside by light, sound, and your complete focused intention. When you finish your fifth sounding of the vowel E into your kidneys, infused with light and intention for ease and wellness, then pause, rest, and breathe.

The Heart and the Vowel I. By now you have established a rhythm with your breath, sounding, and visioning. Take a moment to check in with your body. Give yourself water or a longer pause if needed. Journal if you wish or continue with the ritual and journal afterward.

The heart is a muscle that governs the circulation system, pumping blood around the body, carrying oxygen and nutrients to all parts of the body and waste to be released. In my spirit knowing, the heart is the holder of memory. The rooms or chambers of the heart can become crowded and block entry to new things. We may then resist possibility, as old memories become a barrier, especially if the memories hold harm. Let us sound into your heart now.

Ready yourself with your breath practice, inhaling deeply through your nose and exhaling audibly through your mouth. Place your hand over your beating heart if you are able. Feel the vibration of your heart and breathe. Feel the life energy under your skin. When you are ready, on the exhale sound a long IIIIIIIIIIIIII. Inhale and exhale IIIIIIIIIIII. Then once more, inhale and exhale IIIIIIIIIIIIII, to the end of the breath. Then pause and breathe deeply. Keep your hand and mind on your heart. Notice what rises—images, songs, memories, thoughts. Be curious and witness as you are able. Let the story pass by without leaning into the facts of it; just witness now, please. When you feel ready, bring the imagery of sunlight into your sounding. Imagine sunlight moving on the exhalation, from your breath into your heart, infusing the four chambers of this precious organ with a bright yellow glow. Inhale deeply and exhale IIIIIIIIIIIIII five times into your heart.

As you sound, imagine grief leaving your body, spilling onto the ground like rain cleansing a landscape. When you finish your fifth sounding and visioning, pause and rest. Be with your breath. Check in with yourself. Take care by drinking water, moving, standing, stretching, walking around the room, as you are able. When you are ready, return to a comfortable position.

The Lungs and the Vowel O. Our lungs are pinkish gray organs located on either side of the chest, anchoring the heart on each side. When we inhale, air enters the lungs and oxygen from the air moves through the blood, which provides oxygen and nutrients to the body. Carbon dioxide, a waste gas, moves from the blood to the lungs and is released when we exhale. Grace confirms what my friends who are master practitioners of Traditional Chinese Medicine tell me, that our lungs can hold unlet grief.

Let us sound into your lungs now. Bring your focus to your lungs and place your hands there. Engage your conscious breathing practice. Inhale deeply through your nose and exhale a long OOOOOOOO. Repeat three times. Feel your chest move as you fill your lungs with air and then release completely. After your third exhaling of O, rest for a bit and feel your lungs responding to this practice. Invisible and absolute is air; for many of us, our lungs know how to breathe without our witness or consent.

Imagine now that the air you are inhaling is speckled with colorful light, like glitter tossed high and falling to the ground slowly. Inhale this rainbow light into your lungs through your nose, and exhale through your mouth as you repeat the vowel OOOOOOOOO. Do this five times. Imagine your breath moving through the latticework of tubes and fibers that make up the lungs, gathering anything caught in this framework that does not serve your life. See your lungs able to take in full breaths of fresh, clean air, as you release from your mouth stagnant, old things. When you complete your fifth round of sound and vision, come to quiet and be still. Cycle your breathing as you check in with yourself. Allow your feelings to flow as they wish. Let wherever you are resting support the full weight of your body, and know that the earth is holding you too.

The Pineal Gland and the Vowel U. Guide your awareness, supported by your breath, to your brain. Breathing deeply, consider this organ, seen as an interpreter, initiator, controller, and holder of all our choices. Neuroscientists are in constant, active study of the brain, which is an incredibly complex network with more interconnections than there are stars and planets in the Milky Way. Breathe and consider the great undiscovered gifts housed inside your brain. Grace guides us to the pineal gland, located deep within the center of this incredible organ, behind the space between your eyes. Grace tells me that the pineal gland is indeed our connection to spirit. Imagine this gland, the size of a dried pea, that lets the body know when it is time to rest by the presence of night or morning light.

The pineal gland is the house of our highest knowing of spirit and infinite possibility. Sounding into the pineal gland is like visiting the metaphoric "Upper Room," a sacred place where we commune with our knowing of God, Goddess, Spirit, Divine Love. It is important to hear that all the divinity we honor is also inside us. Cycle your intentional breath practice as you prepare to sound into your brain, focusing on the pineal gland. Imagine the space deep within, behind your eyes. See a small, bright light shining there, like the flame of a candle. See this light as you inhale deeply and exhale UUUUUUUUUU to the end of your breath. Inhale again, and exhale UUUUUUUUUUU. Then again, UUUUUUUUUUUUU. Pause, breathe, and notice.

Hold the vision of light as you prepare to sound five times. Inhale, and exhale UUUUUUUUUU into your brain, toward this steady light. See the light growing as you repeat this practice. When you complete your fifth cycle, come to quiet and notice how you are feeling. Have some water, stretch, move your body a bit by walking around or in place. When you feel ready, return to your position of comfort, and prepare to hum into your pancreas.

The Pancreas and Humming. The pancreas creates natural juices called pancreatic enzymes to break down foods. It is an elongated, pinkish organ nestled under the liver, behind the stomach and in front of your spine. Grace says that the pancreas is where secrets hide, things we are afraid to face, usually connected to intergenerational harm and story. We are bringing voice to the pancreas to uncover and release any energy that does not belong there. Remember: we do not need to understand or even know what harm may have happened to release it. Let us hum into your pancreas.

Begin your breath practice, inhaling deeply through your nose and exhaling audibly through your mouth, as you locate your pancreas and place your hand and mind there as you are able. Imagine this organ, almost hidden from view, resting under your attention. Inhale deeply, and exhale a Hummmmmmm. Again, see your sound full of color-filled light seeping through the pores that cover the skin that covers your pancreas. See your pancreas begin to vibrate from the sound of your voice and the power of your attention. Inhale, and again exhale Hummmmmmm, resting in between, moving slowly to be with anything that may rise in your spirit for your attention—images, narratives, songs, the body has many ways of moving old things. For this practice, hum until you are ready to come to silence. Please trust your body's response. When you finish your humming, lean back and spend some time breathing and resting.

Closing: The Perineum and Humming

We close this ritual the way we opened, by offering gratitude to the ancestors of the land that holds your life and to those that walk beside you. We honor the earth that supports your presence, gives bounty, receives the energy you release from your body and repurposes what you no longer need. Inhaling deeply through your nose and exhaling through your mouth, bring your focus to your perineum. Imagine roots, healthy and strong, descending from this sacred place and moving toward the earth, passing easily through the floor to the soil beneath. See your roots being welcomed by the earth, entering and moving deeper into the ground to settle in soft, moist, dirt. Imagine inhaling from these anchored roots and drawing breath into your body, guiding this breath from root to crown. Inhale deeply and exhale your awareness down your back body, down to the earth again. Bring your voice to this grounding now, inhaling deeply and exhaling your hum five times into your perineum, Hummmmmmmm. Inhale and exhale Hummmmmmmm. Take your time and pause as needed. Exhale Hummmmmmm into the root that begins at your perineum, now living in the earth. Send the vibration of your voice there. Hummmmmmm. And Hummmmmmm to the end of your breath; then inhale and exhale and come to quiet.

Reflection

You did it, family; you have finished this ritual of sounding into your vital organs and humming into your pancreas and perineum. Please take some deep breaths now and feel into what this means. Congratulate yourself. Well done. Take care and make sure you move slowly back into your day. You may notice an immediate shift in how you feel about your voice and your body. Keep checking in with yourself. Notice your energy, thoughts, and capacity. Record your experience of this practice in your journal, so that you may return to it and remember. Ask yourself these questions:

- How are you feeling?

- Was there a moment in the ritual where you felt like you might not continue?

- Did you keep going?

- Was there a particular sound or organ that stood out for you?

- Why?

Please have a good nourishing meal. Get into your medicine bath or shower with a rinse of sea salt and baking soda. Then rest.

You may work with these rituals as you feel guided, sounding through each vital organ or choosing one organ. We encourage you to remember the pineal gland when you pray, to honor divine presence.

Try bringing the pineal gland meditation into your morning practice, visioning the space at the center of your brain vibrating with light and awareness before you move into your day.

7

Sound and Cancer: Caretaking Our Cells

I n January 2019, I received a diagnosis of chronic myeloid leukemia (CML), a rare blood-cell cancer that creates a proliferation of white blood cells in the body. I knew for some time before receiving confirmation that something was happening with my blood. My heart was laboring nightly, as if I was trying to scale a mountain in my sleep. I would wake and sing and talk to my heart, sounding my soul tones to calm my heart and regulate the rhythm. My hair began to thin and then break, so I stepped up my vitamins and changed my diet. I had always been vigilant about getting regular blood work. I have met so many unwell healers and holders of space, and I understand that to channel is to allow infinite energy to move through my finite body. I was attentive to cleaning and releasing energy after holding space in my rituals, and I heard Grace say often that none of us needs to donate any real estate in our body to do our good works. So I was baffled by the news that I had cancer.

And then, I was angry, although pissed off feels like a better description. My ego went off the rails, and I started venting out loud to the universe. My language went something like this:

I am a master healer. How dare y'all bring this to my body?

This is a test? Now I have to heal myself?!

And while ranting at the universe, I noticed the return of a narrative that was born on that doorstep while I watched my mama leave:

No matter what I do, it is never good enough. I can't win.

I felt devastated by this news, and I quickly defaulted to victim consciousness, cloaked in righteous anger. I was particularly angry

123

with Grace. I had no warning that this was going to happen to me, no prophetic dreams, signs, no sudden flashes of precognitive vision. Most of my life I have received advanced intel from spirit around so many things, but not this time.

After days of mourning, I eventually found my way to my prayer practice. I asked my ancestors why this was happening and what was I to do to heal my body. Grace stepped forward and spoke to me about adaptation, about how sometimes what appears to be illness is the body responding and adapting to energies that overwhelm the cells, like too much electric current and not enough wiring. Grace told me that the reasons why would be revealed and that I was to take the medicine offered. I was to follow the protocol set by my doctor for two years, and then I would be able to stop taking the medicine. Grace told me that I would use this walk with cancer to be of deeper service in the world.

Well, family, this is the moment where I get to share again. I am not always a good steward of Grace's instruction. I was indignant and not ready to listen or to follow any directives.

I decided I was going to heal and do it on my own terms, and I turned away from all of my spirit knowing.

Testimony

Before I continue sharing about my experience with cancer, it feels important to say that this is my testimony and not a commentary or judgment on anyone's choices. There is no adequate word to describe the incredible loss that cancer can bring. I only have sound for this grief of missing beloveds whose lives were taken by this disease. And I understand now that writing and telling my story is part of the service Grace spoke of. I have met many healers, leaders, and holders of space who are quietly navigating disease. There is shame and fear around how people will continue to receive their guidance and medicine offerings, as if healers, leaders, and holders of space (or anyone) should be immune and beyond the potential ills of the body. I am not talking about the choice made to keep a diagnosis within a small circle of beloveds. I am talking about those who suffer in silence and metaphorically crawl into dark places. I am talking about myself before I found my way back to my liberation practice. It took me some time to arrive. Here is how I got there.

Leading with Fear

The medicine I was prescribed was an oral chemotherapy, which can make a peson feel nauseous and cause diarrhea and sometimes incontinence. Those who know me well know that I'm a fairly controlling person. Surrender is a full-time practice for me. I did not want to take this medicine. So I didn't. I had no insurance and could not afford to see a specialist, and the physician I was able to see was deeply distracted every time we met, giving me little information and no language around possibility and healing. All I heard was that I must follow the protocol, which was to take the oral chemo for the rest of my life.

I did have enough presence to avoid the rabbit hole of internet research. We are porous beings. I knew that if I read about the symptoms of CML and the side effects of the medicine, I would recreate in my body all that I read. I ignored Grace and the doctor's advice, and I created my own protocol of weekly acupuncture, qigong classes, plant medicine tinctures to strengthen and cleanse the blood, Pilates, power walking, a plant-based diet, lots of water, longer meditations, and no chemo pills. I felt amazing, and for months my blood work showed that I was not getting worse. I was not getting better either. I was hovering in the same place.

In December of 2019, twelve months after the initial diagnosis, I experienced a profoundly painful happening between myself and a friend, which triggered waves of old grief that needed all my attention. I could not sustain my care practice against CML. As I turned toward daily grief-letting and the demands of maintaining my life of music, traveling, holding sound-healing circles, writing, and expanding my practice, my heart began to wake me in the middle of the night again, and my body began to ache.

The first week of January 2020 found me sitting in triage in the emergency room with a body full of pain. A few days before, I had received a call from my daughter, who did not know I had cancer. She had just had a reading with a spiritualist who gave her a message for her mother: "*Tell your mother to stop living in denial. Listen to doctors. Take the medicine.*" Well, this message from spirit only made me angrier. I imagine that some of you are reading this and shaking your head in wonder, and maybe some of y'all can relate. I had not told my daughter about the CML, and I was angry at spirit for violating my privacy. Yes, for real. I am sitting here laughing at myself as I write, humbled by the massive power of the unchecked ego. The truth I could not yet embrace was that I was embarrassed to be sick. I was afraid of how I would be seen and treated, and I did not want my daughter to see me as less than her strong, fierce mama. Anger is usually easier for me to access when I feel shame; it serves the illusion of being powerful and able.

This message from spirit upset my daughter, of course, and we made a date to talk in person. I promised her I would take care and obey this warning. I did not tell her what it was about; instead, I said what needed to be said to soothe her fears. The sound of my daughter's voice full of worry helped break the spell of my resistance. She was about to enter her third trimester. What the hell was I doing, putting myself, and therefore my loves at risk? It was an important moment that brought me to my knees and back to myself.

Three days later I was in the emergency room with a specialist who told me that if I had taken the medicine for two years when I was first diagnosed, there was an excellent chance of the cancer going into remission. Since I had spent so much time working my own protocol, there was a chance now that the medicine would not work as well. The specialist confirmed the information I received initially from Grace.

I left the hospital and began a new protocol that included energy work, plant medicines, meditation rituals, and the prescribed medication. I turned toward the leukemia and began a new relationship with the disease, anchored in acknowledging the present moment, honoring the needs of my body, and visioning my wellness. I began to treat cancer like a guest passing through. I started singing to my blood and imagining my cells vibrant and healed. Whenever I take the medicine, I imagine I am swallowing edible gold that is coating my insides in shimmery light, bringing me gifts, healing my blood. I look down at my skin and imagine gold light filtering through my pores, illuminating the space around my body. I speak words of love to my body and affirm, even as nausea rises, that I am perfect, whole, and well. I affirm that I am in remission, and I believe with all of my being that one day this will be so.

Cancer

Dear family, this is my story, my song about my journey with cancer. I have been privileged to walk beside others as they endeavor to heal from cancer, and each story has been different. Sometimes I have been a death doula on this walk, helping folk leave this realm, and sometimes I have witnessed those in full remission with years of freedom from this disease. I chose to focus this chapter on cancer because of my personal experience working with the diagnosis and treatment and because of the people with cancer who have come to my sound-healing table for guidance and care. Between us, there are shared experiences.

Cancer treatment creates an incredible amount of revenue for pharmaceutical companies and for the physicians who herald one drug over another. The cost of medicines is unsustainable and out of reach for so many. I have felt in my spirit that there is an overarching presence of greed when it comes to treating cancer, through the commodification of grief and fear. The intention for the following rituals is to make anchoring in possibility part of our protocols, to place full attention on loving the parts of our body experiencing disease, to center what is well and healthy and integrate these knowings.

Your Practice Belongs to You

Please know that if you work with the rituals offered below and see minimal change in your body, you are not doing anything wrong. I know these rituals to be of service in myriad ways, shifting perspective about a diagnosis by centering the care of the one who is on the healing journey. This nourishes the spirit and helps keep us buoyed through treatments that deplete the body.

The Sounds We Use, the Words We Choose

I have never used the words "my cancer." I only refer to things that I wish to keep as mine. When first diagnosed, I began to experiment with the phrase "fuck cancer." I completely understood how important it was to move my anger and saying "fuck cancer" felt good and defiant, for a little while. And then it began to make me feel tired. I wondered where the rage was going? If I am saying, "fuck cancer," am I turning this energy against my own body, toward my blood? I began to hold these questions in my spirit and speak them out loud.

I woke one morning hearing that "fuck cancer" shifts our collective rage toward the disease and our bodies, instead of toward horrific systems of oppression and environmental racism that create the conditions that deplete and harm the body and render us vulnerable to illness. I decided to take "fuck cancer" out of my vocabulary. I turn my anger about this disease toward dismantling racism, fascism, poverty, the prison industrial complex, and other forms of violence that nourish disease and cancerous cells. I pray that this offering of rituals be of service to your life as you navigate cancer or other chronic diseases.

—————— Ritual ——————
FOR CARETAKING CANCEROUS CELLS

With this ritual you will be singing to cancerous cells and any part of your body impacted by disease. You may also practice this ritual by listening or tapping a rhythm you find calming into your body. You will use a familiar song or melody and create your own lyrics. Music is a teacher, and we remember the songs we love and absorb the story quickly. When I was a little girl, I learned so much from the video shorts for children in "Schoolhouse Rock"; I passed many a test singing these songs to myself. Use the music from your life. It is already in the fabric of your consciousness.

Tools

- gather your songs

Preparation

Before we begin the practice of caretaking our cells, we want to make sure you are not holding anger in your body around your diagnosis. We do not want anger to be inside of the sound as you sing to your body, as it will bring more harm. Please revisit the ritual to move anger, shared in chapter 3; when you have completed that ritual, please return to this page.

We will be singing, tapping, or playing songs to the parts of your body affected directly by cancer or other disease. Songs of love that bring life-affirming energy only. You will need a half hour or less to complete this ritual. You can work with it throughout the day; try it while doing simple tasks like washing dishes or doing laundry.

My favorite song to use when singing to my blood cells is "You Are So Beautiful" by Billy Preston, a song he wrote for his mother. I grew up listening to this song. It was easy to adapt the melody and change some lyrics to suit my intention. Choose a song and melody that move you and make you feel good. Again, you will be sharing this song to the part of your body impacted by cancer or other disease. I will use the colon as an example.

I made up this song from the lullaby "Twinkle, Twinkle, Little Star":

> *I am singing to my bones*
> *cause my body is my home*
> *and I love my colon strong.*
> *It does good work the whole day long.*
> *My digestion works for me,*
> *and my colon is healthy*

This practice is not about being a singer. It is about your intention and practice of loving on a part of your body that needs your care.

Ritual

You do not need to begin this ritual from a place of meditation. You can start anytime. While singing, listening, or tapping the song you have chosen to the part of your body with cancer, imagine the song and vibration landing on your skin, seeping through your pores, eventually to rest on disease in your body. Imagine and see your intention of care going where you send it, circling the place in need, and bringing grace there. If this feels difficult, pause and take three deep, conscious breaths. Now think of someone or something you love. Recall this energy and sing, listen, or tap from this place of remembering love. Consider the well cells and organs in your body and send light there too. Imagine your whole being lit from within with the sound and vibration of your voice and intention, sourced from a sense of well-being and love.

Closing

We do not close this ritual. I sing to my blood daily, and I invite you to work with this ritual daily too. Wherever you are, whatever you are doing, you may practice this at anytime. After a while, you will be caretaking your cells all the time, in the shower, while driving, food shopping, riding public transportation—it will become part of your daily routine. You won't need to focus on the part of the body with disease; your body memory will hold the intentions you have set.

―――――――――― Ritual ――――――――――

TO PREPARE FOR SURGERY

I had a client who had breast cancer. They are now in full remission. They had a double mastectomy to completely remove both breasts. Here is the ritual we worked with to prepare for surgery.

Preparation

My client would engage this practice every morning for fifteen minutes, as soon as they woke, before leaving their bed. If you are able, this is a great time for this ritual.

Ritual

Begin with bringing your full awareness to your breath. Inhale deeply through your nose, and exhale slowly through your mouth. As you feel able, relax your body. Bring your awareness and your breath to your shoulders and work your way down your spine. Journey around your body while cycling your breath. Notice your feelings and name your feelings as you breathe. For example:

> *I am afraid.*
> *I am sad.*
> *I am grateful.*
> *I allow myself to feel all my feelings.*

Give voice to what rises in your body. Then, turn your attention to the part of your body that will be altered or changed by surgery, and place your hands there if you are able. Touch the closest area approximate to where the surgeons will enter to do their work. My client would place a hand over each breast. Imagine the area under your hands full of light. Place your full attention there and begin to speak this mantra to your body, out loud if you can:

> *I love you, body; you are beautiful and mine.*
> *As my body changes, it is still beautiful and mine.*

Name the part of your body that will be operated on, and love this part by name.

Closing

Close your ritual to prepare for surgery with this affirmative prayer. Speak in the present tense, as if what you are praying on has already happened:

I am grateful for the success of my surgery. I am healing under grace.
I bless the hands and hearts of all those involved in my care. I
am well.
All is well.

Visit this prayer throughout your day. If fear rises, turn to look at it. Acknowledge that it is present for you, and then greet this fear with your prayer.

——— Affirmations ———
FOR BEING IN REMISSION

You may work with these affirmations at any point in your treatment. Use the words as you vision your wellness, as a way of calling to you what you wish to receive, and when you are in remission, to hear yourself claim your present moment of healing. Say these affirmations to yourself during your morning practice or throughout your day, as you wish.

- My body is free from cancer. I am cancer free.
- I feel love inside of the medicines I take; love heals my body through this medicine.
- I am breathing life. My cancer-free body loves a deep breath, and I am loving my body by breathing.
- Cancer did not come to stay. I am healed. It went away.
- My body is my sanctuary. I own all of it.
- My body is my sanctuary, even though I was sick.
- My body is my spirit home; peace lives here too. I am not alone.
- My body is my sanctuary, and I love living well.

Ritual

FOR PRESENCE

Living Day to Day with Cancer and Other Diseases

The following ritual is a practice of presence, of staying inside each moment. Some diagnoses predict when we will die, and in my experience, these dates are never real. I have witnessed people live far beyond the expected time line, grateful they did not stop engaging with life. As a woman of spirit, I have always thought of death as a doorway to another realm, just as important as the realm that holds my living, breathing body. I am not afraid to die, and I don't want to leave my children and my grandchildren and all those I love. Receiving a cancer diagnosis caused me to consider my mortality, and I decided that I would deepen my relationship with living.

I became more intentional with every breath, taste, touch, and sound. I do more seeing and less looking. When I am not holding space, I try to talk less and listen more to people and everything. There are (not so) hidden messages everywhere, guiding us. And though I absolutely vision holding my great grandchildren in my arms, I know that there may be a different plan for me, one I do not control. So I do not live in the fearful place of what may happen. I revel in the moment to moment of all that I choose.

Here is a simple ritual that helps us practice being present with the moment we are living, by eating, tasting, and savoring something wonderful.

Tools

- your favorite healthy treat (for me it is rich dark chocolate)

Preparation

Please choose the sweet, savory, sour, or bitter taste that brings you joy. Mine are coffee and dark chocolate. I will use dark chocolate as an example.

Ritual

Hold a small piece of your favorite chocolate and lean forward to inhale the fragrance. Place the chocolate on your tongue. Savor it; do not chew. Close your mouth over the chocolate and take a deep, slow breath. Notice how the fragrance tastes as it begins to melt on your tongue. Move your tongue so that the chocolate is sandwiched between it and the roof of your mouth. Notice the flavors. Do you taste cinnamon or vanilla? Swallow then and notice the feeling and taste at the back of your throat. Breathe and savor.

Closing

I offer no closing to this ritual. Please savor everything wonderful, daily. See the sky, notice light, dark, inhale beauty. Feel the weight and blessing of water in your mouth when you drink, on your skin when you bathe, and in your hands when it rains. Consider the night sky, the wonders that lie beyond all that is seen. Have another piece of chocolate or bite or sip of your chosen treat. The point is to revel. Most of us do not know when we will be invited to leave this realm, or how. We do know that infinite time on earth is not promised to us. When we revel, we are showing love to ourselves and sharing love too, as this energy will be palpable to everyone around us. I wish you many moments of love and ease for the difficult journey of living with disease. I hold the knowing of the healing that is possible. May it be so.

part four

SOUNDING
— *into the* —
WORLD

this is a song about coming together
this is a song about how
word I am word and I know how to serve,
this is a song about now
somebody told us to love one another
quiet the mind and be still—
now is the time to believe who we are, and
marry your soul with your will—
cause we are the ones who will heal,
now is the time to believe who you are, remember, only love is real.

8

Sound and Language Justice: Multilingual Grace

Dear family, English is not Grace's first language. Sometimes they will speak through me using their language, and I understand the words as I hear them leaving my mouth. Then the meaning will leave my consciousness, though the feeling of what was said remains in my body. Grace's language has a steady cadence and sound that reminds me of old recordings I've heard of the Powhatan tribe, Indigenous Algonquian people from eastern Virginia. I believe this language is no longer spoken. It is beautiful to me, and I love when Grace uses my voice to speak in their tongue. I am often asked if I am "speaking in tongues," which I associate with my grandmother's church in Apalachicola. "Tongues" is known to be a divine expression from God that comes through a person who is experiencing possession by the Holy Spirit. Grace's language feels like it comes from a lineage that has no experience of colonization. There are many sounds (words) for love and none that express separation, otherness, war, loss, or harm. Everything is one thing; all beings are one being. When this language comes through me, I feel an overwhelming sense of clarity and something akin to simplicity. I am clear in those moments that only love is real.

Our Language Is Who We Be

In this chapter, I share an experience that transformed my relationship with the English language and provided more evidence of the healing that can happen when we greet each other with curiosity and respect.

In the fall of 2020, I was invited to bring sound-healing rituals to the organization Move to End Violence (MEV), a capacity-building and leadership development program for US leaders working to end gender-based violence. I was privileged to work with this incredible circle of people for two years, learning from the brilliance and presence of those shepherding and holding the organization and from the powerful commitment and love of the movement makers invited to join the program. While working with MEV, I was introduced to the practice of "language justice" as a framework for social change, inclusion, healing, and liberation. I learned of organizations that have been leading this work for many years. It was revelatory and humbling for me to realize how much I did not understand about power dynamics and language, who gets to be heard and therefore seen, honored, cared for, and known.

As I became available to this learning, Grace spoke to me of the generational devastation caused by the criminalization and erasure of languages and the loss of ancestral languages due to a multitude of horrors and dispossession. I became a student in the practice of language justice because of my time with the MEV community. The efficacy of their work and commitment to creating an environment where all peoples across race, gender, sexual orientation, ability, class, region, and dialect have opportunity and equal access showed me what a practice of solidarity looks like in real time and what is possible for our interwoven, multilingual communities.

Sound, Interpretation, Healing

With MEV, I had my first experience of offering sound healing and spiritual guidance to people who speak languages other than my own. The expertise of profoundly gifted interpreters allowed these offerings to happen and our medicine to be shared. We were able to work with many people in this way. Here is the story of one session that continues to bless and lift my spirit.

Through most of the beginning years of COVID-19, I was privileged to be able to offer my work virtually. My return to working in person happened with MEV in the spring of 2022, for a large convening of activists and movement makers. Part of my responsibility was to offer morning meditation and to help participants ground in the day's intention. On the first morning, I was approached by an Afro-Indigenous organizer from Central America, who with the aid of an interpreter, told me that as soon as they heard my voice, they remembered dreaming about me the night before they traveled to this gathering. They shared that their spirit guides told them I would help them release old wounds and sadness from their body. They asked if they could work with me. We scheduled a session, and I requested two interpreters I felt deeply connected to for support, who both agreed to co-hold the session.

We met the next day. The three of us circled my client as I lay hands on their body and toned and placed sound into their skin, speaking prayers from Grace that were translated with great care by the interpreters. We worked in this way for a while, me praying and toning into organs and chakras and the interpreters channeling the perfect words in the beloved's native language. It was a deep, potent ritual of multilingual grace. The interpreters brought their own medicine, which was felt in their sound as they took turns sharing our instructions and prescriptions for reclamation and renewal. My client responded to our offering by releasing much grief and sharing some of their story. I was able to hear and feel the sound of their voice as the interpreters guided me in English. We closed the session with words of love and healing, which are palpable beings that know no boundaries. The client thanked us and left the room shining brightly from within and feeling freer.

Inspired by language justice practitioners, I began a daily practice of dismantling my sense of entitlement as an English-speaking person born in the United States. I was weaned on the untruth that English is the chosen language of the world community. This thought is a stealthy one that requires vigilance and patience to uproot in my being. I am committed to learning Spanish so that I can converse with some of my closest friends who spoke Spanish before learning English. I know I will discover more about them when I am able to speak to them in the language of the mothers of their mothers. These friends have also shared with me the emotional complexities that come with speaking a language that was weaponized with the intent to eradicate Indigenous cultures and peoples around the globe. We hold the knowing of this harm alongside our intention to build connection, and we use our language to create bridges.

The language justice movement is integral to all anti-oppression and liberation work.

Please see "Recommended Resources" in this book to discover organizations and collectives that are leading this good work. There are many people working on behalf of our interwoven multilingual communities, teaching us how to honor and embrace each other as we are. Another example among them is "queering," which challenges heteronormativity, gender, sexuality, identity politics, and systems of oppression with language that removes all traces of gender violence, oppression, and harm.

——————— Practice ———————

CONNECTION

Collectively, there are more than seven thousand languages spoken in the world today, and more than three hundred different sign languages. To engage this practice, you will need to download a translation application to your smartphone. Also do some research on a computer or choose books that offer general language learnings and hone in on a particular language you wish to learn. Use all these tools whenever you are communicating with someone whose language of origin is different from your own, especially if English is your first language. Do not assume that the person you are speaking with should speak English too. Ask them if you may try some simple exchanges using their mother tongue and then do your best using your translator. I have found that people feel seen and will appreciate your efforts, even when you get it wrong. Connection happens, usually with laughter and good feelings.

We have the opportunity to stand in each other's humanity and learn something about each other.

If you live in a place where you do not often encounter people who speak other languages, take some time to sit at a computer and find your way to people speaking, singing, and signing in different languages. Is there a language that you've always been curious about? Try listening to several different dialects to see if your spirit responds to one or the other. Watch movies with English subtitles or the language you are most comfortable with. Go to your local library to find books that will introduce you to foods, customs, and practices of people from around the globe. Decide to learn about the myriad ways of communicating. Be curious and be guided by what calls to you.

Ritual

FOR COMMON HUMANNESS
People Who Need People

Here is a practice that can help us see our common humanity and release any untruths that cause us to engage in othering.

Tools

- movies with subtitles you can easily read
- a timer
- a journal

Preparation

Choose three movies with a common theme from three different countries, or choose a film that includes ASL (American Sign Language) or another country's sign language. Plan to watch all three movies, engaging the subtitles, over seven days. I recommend something sweet and lighthearted, like a romantic comedy or intergenerational fun. Prepare your snacks, and make yourself comfortable as you get ready to enjoy the film. Note the length of time for your movie, and set your timer for half that time.

Practice

As you begin to watch, pay close attention to the subtitles as you listen to the voices of the characters. When your timer chimes, turn off the subtitles. Now, listen to the voices and watch the faces and body language of the actors in the second half of the film. After the movie, open your journal and answer these questions:

- Did you connect with any of the characters in the movie?

- Did anyone in the movie remind you of someone you know?

- Did you recognize the story? Did it feel familiar?

- Did any of the characters remind you of yourself?

Watch the other two films before the end of the week in the same way: turn off the subtitles midway through the movie, and after the movie, journal your answers to the same questions.

Closing

The intention of this practice is to recognize how very human we are. There are many things that make us different, and many things that make us same. We all need love. We need food, shelter, care, fresh water, and clean air. We want our children and our loves to be safe and well. We all bleed, breathe, and have hearts that beat, a constant vibration that signals aliveness. Speaking different languages is a fake barrier to knowing each other better. We invite you to learn all you can about the peoples of the world. It is not hyperbole when we say we need each other. We need each other.

9

Sound and Climate Change:
Us Holding Our World

n the 1970s, summer fun in Brooklyn was an open fire hydrant. All the
kids on the block would show up to play, and we would hang out by
the curb, dodging cars and running through the cool water. We would
spend whole days in Prospect Park, playing with marbles in dirt, climbing
trees, rolling down hills, and trying to fish in the lake with poles we made
from sticks, string, and paper clips. Sometimes my father would take us
to Coney Island to hang out on the boardwalk or to Brighton Beach. My
father would pay his fare and wait on the train platform. When we heard
the train coming, my siblings and I would jump over or climb under the
turnstile and run onto the D train just as the doors were closing. We got
ices at the beach with our train fare, and the trade always felt worth the risk.

I loved summer. My birthday coincided with the last day of school,
a double celebration. My siblings' birthdays are in late fall and winter; I
was the lucky one. Summers in my Brooklyn were full of block parties,
fireworks, and sleeping on the fire escape because we had no air con-
ditioning. We played outside in the heat all day long, tracking the sun,
willing time to move slower. We knew that as soon as the sun dipped
below the horizon, the streetlights would come on and it would be time
to go home. Life for me and many of my friends was always sweeter
outside. Home was synonymous with ongoing trauma. We had that in
common. Summers brought respite, and sunlight was salvation.

My love affair with summer days shifted in my fifth-grade science class.

Our teacher told us a terrifying story about a hole in the earth's atmo-
sphere that put us all at risk for something called skin cancer. He told

us that we needed to go home and tell our parents to stop using aerosol cans so we could save the environment. We learned new words that day, *stratosphere, ozone layer,* and *global warming.* I remember feeling angry with my teacher. I wanted grown-ups to take care of this new problem. My ten-year-old takeaway was that now I had to be wary of sunlight.

Dear family, I am a grandmother now. I am one of the grown-ups who must caretake this problem. In just 47 summers, we have edged closer to what climatologists call a "climate tipping point." Tipping past that point leads to irreversible and potentially catastrophic effects on the world's ecosystems. We are already inside the effects of climate change, and we can still take action. We have the tools to limit further damage and strategies to adapt to where we are standing now. Climate change is a complex issue, mostly driven by choices rooted in greed, made by those who also protect themselves from the devastation of so-called "natural disasters." There is nothing natural about flooding caused by deforestation or contaminated drinking water due to mountaintop removal. Generations of people who make a living from mining and those of us who depend on coal are inside a reckoning, and we all play a part, as there are no small gestures here.

Every choice we make matters, from how we travel to the food we eat, the electricity we use, and what we do to help those whose lives and livelihoods are immediately affected by environmental calamity. For many of us, our response to this present moment, where we stand on the precipice of climate disaster, is fear and an inability to turn fully toward the reality of what is happening. We feel overwhelmed, so we send prayers and money to the country, city, or town affected by the latest weather-driven hardship, and we hope that *something* will save us.

We are the ones who will heal. Money and prayers are important forms of energy. We want to support the organizations doing the daily work of addressing climate change and climate justice. Climate justice is a global social movement exposing the injustice that those who bear the least responsibility for climate change are suffering the most. Activists pressure governments and industry to find solutions to the climate crisis and care for those most impacted. (You will find a list of organizations doing the work on climate change and climate justice near the end of this book, in "Recommended Resources.")

And the earth is asking us to do more. We must radically shift our relationship with how we use our natural resources: water, oil, gas, metals, coal, electricity, wind, solar power, and the power of our life force, our chi. There are new technologies that will support the deeply difficult walk of weaning ourselves from fossil fuels and monitoring our carbon footprint. We can be better stewards of the earth and learn to accept the fact that climate change is already in play. And we must make every effort to be of service to the children of our children.

As we deepen our daily practice on our personal healing journey, all beings benefit from how we are learning to take care of ourselves. The patient, loving regard we give to ourselves and our beloveds, we can learn to share as well with the earth and all its inhabitants. Our rituals of grief-letting, soul retrieval, and witnessing can create in us a deeper capacity to face the things we fear. It is our liberation practice that allows us to turn our full attention and power to shifting climate change.

What we do to others, we do to ourselves—this is spiritual law. I will add that what we do to the environment, we are doing to ourselves. Let those of us who can begin to take full control of the choices we govern. We don't need every person on the planet to practice conservation. We need a critical mass of folk in shared agreement, and this is beginning to happen.

One practice on this journey of restoring ecological balance is to release the illusion of separation and honor the irrefutable fact that all life is interdependent. Please say this out loud to yourself right now:

All Life Is Interconnected.

Feel how these words land in your spirit. What do you think about this concept? Say it again, please, and repeat it to yourself for a few minutes. Notice your body's response. Be curious. How does it make you feel? If this is true, what does it mean for how you live?

We begin this practice to restore balance in our present moment, wherever we are living. Actions that may feel like small steps are vital. All that we do to correct the course of climate change makes a difference to the whole. We are to practice simultaneity: acknowledging the challenges of this moment while also holding the vision of what we want and doing the work to make it happen. Let us imagine a critical mass of people in shared agreement of what is still possible for the healing of our planet, and let it begin with you and me.

WALKING MEDITATION
Ritual
I Breathe the Earth, the Earth Breathes Me

This is a walking meditation that may be practiced in a park, on the beach, by a river, in the woods or any natural setting. Please adapt this offering to your accessibility needs, any movement outside is fine. If you can't be outside, sit comfortably where you are and imagine that you are reveling in nature. The intention of this ritual is to support you in embracing your connection to the natural world, as you connect these words with your movement, speaking aloud and planting this truth inside your body.

Preparation

Memorize this practice if you can. You will be speaking the words aloud, leaning into the sound and vibration of your voice. You are welcome to record this ritual or to write it on a separate piece of paper to hold in your hand as you walk. And be mindful of what is around you.

Ritual

Bring your awareness to your breath as you slowly inhale through your nose and exhale through your mouth; cycle this practice. When you feel ready, in between breaths, begin to say these words softly to yourself:

> *I inhale the sky; I exhale the ground.*
> *I inhale the sky; I exhale the ground.*
> *I inhale the sky; I exhale the ground.*

Feel the ground beneath your body, supporting your walk or your sit. Glance at the sky above you, or imagine its beauty and vastness. Are there clouds, birds, stars, rain? What is your sky doing? See or imagine, and continue speaking out loud:

> *I inhale the sky. I exhale the ground.*
> *I inhale the sky; I exhale the ground.*
> *I inhale the sky; I exhale the ground.*

Notice what you notice: people, pets, green grass, red dirt; autumn, summer, spring, or winter weather, the sounds around you, the feel of wet grass, dry leaves, the wind across your skin. Notice or imagine as you breathe deeply and slowly, inhaling through your nose and exhaling through your mouth. When you are ready, say to yourself:

> *My voice is powerful and pristine, like the mighty headwaters*
> *of the Amazon, Mississippi, Alabama, Yangtze, and all the*
> *rivers of the earth.*
> *My veins and arteries carry life's blood like the roots of Oak,*
> *Baobab, Cypress, Tupelo, and all the trees of the earth.*
> *My heart anchors my life like a taproot that descends to the center*
> *of rock, iron, ore, diamond, and all the minerals of the earth.*
> *My lungs breathe me, generous and deep, like rainforests*
> *breathe for all the creatures of the earth.*
> *My eyes release tears like rain cleansing and nourishing the*
> *land; water is vital to all beings of the earth.*
> *My skin holds my body, a dwelling for my soul, like the ocean*
> *floor and the mountaintop; the earth holds all things.*
> *I Am, we are, all life is one life.*
> *I Am, we are, all life is one life.*
> *I Am, we are, all life is one life.*

This meditation on oneness may be engaged as often as you wish. Imagine what you are saying as you speak the words. See trees, rivers, rainforests, an ocean floor, and mountaintops in your mind's eye, and feel your heart beating and your body breathing. Listen to the sound of your voice and practice speaking these words in a calm, soothing way, the way you speak when you seek to bring comfort to someone. The vibration of your voice, wrapped in the intention of peace, can bring a feeling of connection with the world that surrounds you.

Closing

You close your walking meditation by turning toward the rest of your day. We invite you to cycle the words *I Am, we are, all life is one life* often, to allow this knowing to become part of your everyday thinking. *Audio recordings of these practices are available at soundstrue.com/vibration-of-grace-bonus.

—————— Daily Practices ——————
WAKING TO PRESENCE

Here are simple rituals you may practice daily, as able, that may expand our awareness of nature:

- Greet trees as you pass them on the road; admire their majesty and thank them for the gift of fresh air, shade, fruit, and myriad medicines.

- When you feel the wind on your skin, exhale and imagine that the wind is gifting you with an energetic cleansing, taking all that you are releasing and repurposing.

- When you feel the sun on your face, remember that life on earth is possible because of the sun's light, heat, and energy.

- Notice patterns in nature, a language of interconnection that is everywhere present. Pay attention. Riverbeds throughout our planet look like veins and arteries in the body, carrying fresh water across the earth the way blood is carried to the heart and lungs. The path of the vagal nerves in the body, moving inexorably toward the pelvic floor, looks like the roots of trees moving toward the center of the earth. Spirals, circles, hexagons, fractals, repeated shapes in nature. What will you discover about the earth and yourself once you take a closer look?

- Watch birds in flight. Imagine the bird's view from the sky, of you and all that surrounds you. Take to the air for a moment and look down. What do you see? Imagine feeling a sense of expansion, and take deeper, slower breaths to allow this feeling to take hold of your being.

——————— It's Time ———————

PRACTICE FOR MOVING FROM PASSIVE TO ACTIVE

Here is information that may guide you to a deeper understanding of climate change and teach you what steps you can take to slow or stop the progression of climate disaster. We'll share a couple of ideas here to start you off:

1. We invite you to watch these two videos to educate yourself and learn real-time solutions. There are many videos available that address these topics. I chose these two for the clarity of explanation and solutions offered:

- *The Race Is On: Secrets and Solutions of Climate,* produced by Global Documentary (2019)

- "The fastest way to slow climate change now," a TED Countdown Talk by Ilissa Ocko (2022)

Both videos can be found on the global online video platform Youtube.com. Take some time to watch them, and then write down any questions you may have in your journal.

2. Another option is to go through the list of organizations connected to climate justice and climate change we provide in "Recommended Resources" at the back of this book. Do your research and learn and decide which you will follow, join, or support. The literature from these organizations will probably have answers to some of your questions. Find out what you can do in your home, neighborhood, city, to be more involved with this movement. Here are a few simple things you can do with potentially big impact:

- Unplug all appliances and devices after charging.

- Consider an electric car

- Research clean energy sources, and share your findings.

- Find a group of like-minded and intentioned folk and subscribe to their newsletter and look for ways to participate.

Remember: do not measure your reach against the need; do what is yours to do.

———————— Rituals ————————

FOR TAKING YOURSELF OUT
OF THE FIRE AND FLOOD

These rituals of reclamation can help release fear and resistance, which can take hold of the body when we experience the terror of being in a fire or flood that destroys property, damages the landscape, and takes life. These rituals create the conditions for you to take yourself out of the perpetual harm of reenacting what happened. Living through what I believe are "unnatural disasters" (disasters that are the result of or worsened by humans living without regard for ecological balance) can make it painfully difficult to reconnect with nature and can cause us to feel like the earth is angry with us and being retaliatory. It is a difficult practice, not taking nature's response to global warming personally. This is something to consider: climate disaster is not an act of retribution but an organic response to imbalance. This knowledge can help shift our focus from protecting ourselves from the earth's wrath, which can make us constrict and anchor in separation, to seeing ourselves as firmly part of the whole and able to effect change, which gives us an experience of expansion and curiosity.

The following rituals are practiced in the imaginal realm. You will return to each fear-filled happening and guide yourself to a safe place, saying incantations to encircle yourself and seal the moment. You may need to engage in the rituals more than once. As you begin to practice, please check in with your body and notice how you are feeling. Take your time and stay with your breath practice as you are able. Be gentle and kind with yourself; know that you may pause or stop these rituals as you may need.

Out of the Fire

I have dear friends who have lost their homes to wildfires in California. This ritual was created to serve their healing. May this be so for anyone who has suffered because of a fire.

Tools

- two candles, can be seven-day candles (one orange and one white) and matches

- a fireplace or a fire pit

- a journal

Preparation

If you have a fireplace or fire pit you will not need to use candles, and you may use both if you wish. Choose a quiet place where you will not be disturbed. Sit or lie comfortably, allowing your back body to be supported completely. Soften or close your eyes, and slowly bring your awareness to your breath. Inhale deeply through your nose, and exhale slowly through your mouth. Focus on cycles of this breath for as long as you wish. Once your body begins to feel at rest, stay with your breath practice as you remember the place and time of the fire you experienced.

Ritual

From the safety of your present moment of rest and breath, turn to the memory of the fire that may have taken precious things and displaced your life. Remember and recall. Inhaling deeply through your nose and exhaling through your mouth, feel your back body, lean deeper into the pillows or couch or wherever you're resting and allow yourself to be supported. Turning your attention to the fire, where are you? Are you inside of a home or outside watching? Are you on the express-way trying to get clear of trees and brush burning alongside the road? Feel into your back body and deepen your breath, inhaling slowly and exhaling slowly. From this place of rest and support, imagine yourself beside the you who is dealing with fear and fire.

Speak to yourself out loud, and call yourself by name. Tell yourself you will be safe, and then guide yourself out of the moment. If you are outside watching, imagine leading yourself away. If you are inside trying to get out, lead yourself out. Get yourself well beyond the reach of the fire and care for yourself. Witness yourself. Speak words of care to the one who was just rescued and tell yourself you are safe.

When you are ready, open your eyes. If you have a fireplace or a fire pit, bring your journal and prepare to light a fire. If you do not, prepare to light your two candles, placing them in front of you on a table or a nightstand. As you prepare to light your fire, say some words that honor this elemental:

I see the power of fire and how it can bring warmth, light, and protection.

Once in front of the contained fire, lean into your breath work and rest your eyes on the flames. Focus on inhaling deeply through your nose and holding the breath for about three seconds, then exhale audibly through your mouth. Do this breath five times. With your eyes resting on the flame, consider the fire and feel into your body's response. Write down what you discover. Here are some questions to ask yourself:

- Is it difficult to sit with fire?
- Am I afraid?
- Am I angry about what happened?
- Am I sad?

Answer these questions and add anything you wish, then return to gazing at the flames.

Bring your voice to the moment if you are able, by humming softly to yourself as you consider the answers you gave to the questions. Send your hum around your body, to your stomach, the base of your throat, to any place where your body may need attention. Notice if you are feeling any grief. If you feel tears rising in your body, give this grief to the fire by crying with sound, and imagine that you are directing your grief to the flames. When you feel ready, inhale deeply and exhale audibly three times. Then recite to yourself:

> *I bless and release everything that fire has taken.*
> *I work with fire in controlled and thoughtful ways.*
> *Fire can bring renewal; fire can be of service.*
> *I am present and able to heal from all that has happened.*

Open your journal and write down your answers to these questions:

- How are you feeling?
- Was this ritual of service to you?
- Why?

Include anything else you wish to record, and sit in front of the fire as long as you wish.

Closing

Make sure that your fire is put out completely; blow out your candles as well. If you wish to leave your candles burning, place each one in a bowl of water and set it in a safe place. Over the next few days, check in with yourself by turning your thoughts toward the fire and noticing how these thoughts land in your body. Do you feel any distance or sense of relief? Are you feeling less or no more fear?

Out of the Flood

In September 2021, Hurricane Ida caused incredible amounts of rainfall across the Northeast. In New York City, my daughter was putting my grandson to bed when water began to pour into the living room of her apartment, located just below street level. Flooding happened quickly, and she found herself wading through hip-deep water, trying not to panic so her toddler would not be afraid. She and so many of her neighbors were frightened, trying to gather what they could and get to higher ground. Flooding is the most common unnatural disaster happening in the US, displacing whole communities, creating profoundly stressful conditions that can cause anxiety, depression, and PTSD. I will share that our family was privileged to have access to places where my daughter and grandson could go to be safe and protected from the storm. We know that many, many people do not have this option.

This ritual will help move grief and fear from your body caused by flooding in your home or community. My daughter's relationship to water shifted after her experience. The sound of a hard rain could bring a feeling of nervousness—a quite common response. This offering is designed for you to restore or reclaim your relationship with rain, rivers, and oceans, by bringing the comfort that being in water can give to the memory of harm.

Tools

- a bathtub or a shower
- a journal

- sea salt

- a pitcher of drinking water and a large glass

- warm, soft, comfortable clothes and socks

- a weighted or heavy blanket

- the sound of thunder, oceans, streams, rain

Preparation

Open your journal and record your thoughts as you consider how water is essential to all life on Earth. An adult human body is about 60 percent water (hydrating with water is crucial to a healthy body). Think and write about your relationship with water the day before your experience with flooding and then the day after. Notice any difference. Answer these questions:

- Was safe drinking water available in your area after you survived the flooding?

- Is the water in your community safe to drink now?

- Have you been able to return to your home?

- How do you feel about rain now, and what happens in your body when you see rain in the forecast?

Answer these questions and include anything else you wish to record.

When you finish journaling, find the sound of the ocean, river, or rain online (perhaps at Youtube.com), or you can use a sound machine, an app on your phone, or another audio recording. Make sure the sound you choose will not be interrupted by ads; you will be playing the soundtrack softly in the background for the first part of your ritual.

Read through the ritual before you begin, and take as long as you need to complete this. Once you have read through the entire practice, you can work with this ritual in parts, as needed.

Ritual

We recommend you do this ritual as close to bedtime as possible. Begin by turning on the ocean, river, or rain sounds, and lie down on your back, if you can. Place a pillow under your knees for support, and cover your body with a weighted or heavy blanket. Make sure you feel comfortable. Turn your thoughts toward your breath; inhale slowly through your nose and exhale audibly through your mouth. As you feel your body begin to relax, guide your mind to remembering your experience of flooding. Imagine you are watching this moment as you feel your body supported, held by where you are resting, and know that you are safe as you remember and witness yourself.

Practice inhaling slowly and exhaling slowly, as you recall what happened, how you felt, and how you responded to water rising around you. Witness, remember, stay conscious of your breath. If you begin to feel anxious, steady yourself by pausing and turning your full focus to your breath. When you feel calmer, return to remembering. Bring your calm and steady present moment of breathwork to the memory of flood waters rising. You know you will make it to safety. Bring this knowing to the memory as you recall how you were able to leave or move to higher ground.

Once you have moved through your memory and are safely away from the flooding, slowly bring your awareness to your body, resting. Open your eyes, rise, and gather your warm and comfortable clothes, your glass and pitcher of water, and bring these things into your bathroom. Prepare to take a bath or shower. You may turn off the sound or let it play softly in the other room. Do not add any medicines to this bath or shower, and do not use soap. Sit in a tub full of water, lean back, close your eyes, and rest. Feel the weight of water on your body. If you are in the shower, feel the water on your body. Close your eyes, and bring your awareness to your breath. Imagine you are washing the flood waters from your skin, again.

While soaking or showering, close your eyes and bring your voice to this ritual. Ask the water to draw the moment of memory and the flood waters from your pores. Bring your awareness to your body and give yourself permission to release. Remember the brown flood waters rising, how your body moved through this water, as you continue to inhale slowly and deeply and exhale audibly. If grief rises during this practice, please allow your tears to flow into the bath or shower, and give this grief sound if you can. When you feel it is time, leave the water and drain the tub. If you have been sitting in the tub, take a quick shower to rinse your body of any residue energy. Pour a bit of sea salt into your tub or shower drain; this keeps the energy of the memory moving.

Dress in your warm comfy clothes, and pour yourself a clear glass of water from your pitcher. Hold your glass up to your mouth and pray audibly into the water before drinking. You can use my prayer or create your own:

> *I bless this water. May it move through my body with ease.*
> *May it carry nutrients and oxygen to my cells. May it merge*
> *with my blood*
> *and nourish my beating heart.*

Sip the water and follow the course of the flow, as it passes your lips, over your tongue, to your throat, and down to your stomach, where it will be absorbed by your small intestine into your bloodstream. Excess water will be processed by your kidneys and released from your body.

Closing

Journal about your experience of the ritual. Write whatever comes to mind. Allow a period of freewriting, and do not check what you've written. Choose an affirmation from the list offered in chapter two and cycle this affirmation before bed or throughout your day. After a few days, open your journal and turn to your memory of the flood. Notice your body's response. Ask and record your answers now to these questions:

- Do you feel that the ritual of taking yourself out of the flood served you?

- Why?

- Does the memory of your experience have the same effect on you now?

Then read what you wrote in your journal after completing the ritual, and notice what may have shifted. Record this in your journal.

———— Affirmation Ritual ————
HEALING THE BODY, HEALING THE EARTH

Family, there is nothing linear about how we heal. We practice, make progress, and return to the beginning to practice again. Sometimes this walk of healing feels circular, sometimes sideways and backward. And we keep doing the work for ourselves and our beloveds. Let us affirm that we will do our part to heed the earth's call and use our collective power to bring forth the changes that need to happen to ensure a future of sweet summer days for our babies. Let's give our grandchildren's children the opportunity to be with the incredible beauty of this planet by doing our work today.

We will be in shared agreement and say this affirmation out loud daily:

> *I do everything in my power to ensure that our beautiful planet will endure.*
> *I Am a protector of fresh water, oceans, and air; I honor trees and life everywhere.*

If you will hold this affirmation and join me as I release these words of prayer-filled knowing into the invisible all and the inexhaustible energy of love. Please close this moment with words from your tradition or close as I do by saying, "Ashe, Amen, and so it is."

Conclusion

Sound and a New World:
Wake Up ErrBody

Beloved family, we have come to the end of this book. Thank you for your presence. From my heart to your heart, I wish you daily joy. Please continue to embrace these offerings as you feel called, and take good, good care of yourselves. I have learned that caring for myself will be a lifelong, ever evolving journey that will take many forms. Sometimes it is the simple pleasure of turning my face toward sunlight; other days it is me rising an hour before my household wakes to sit quietly and meditate or do nothing. These acts allow me to pause and replenish my energy reserves, and I cherish every moment. To pause is to Presence Awareness Using Sacred Expression. Breathing is a sacred act, and something all beings have in common. The body loves a deep breath, so please gift yourself moments of deep breathing often throughout your day.

My dear friend, mentor, and ancestor Sekou Sundiata used to say to me that we are living in *all of a sudden times*, meaning that life is moving very quickly everywhere, with no time to prepare. In my Brooklyn, we had a saying for emergent events, *If you stay ready you don't have to get ready*. Daily practice prepares us for the ever-changing world around us. Our rituals for healing, expansion, and release will keep us present. Daily practice helps us to stay ready. There is a new world coming and we get to shape it and decide what it will be. May it be rooted in love and liberation. May all beings know Grace.

We thank you for bringing your vibration, sound, and attention to *The Vibration of Grace* and allowing us to be of service. Bless you as you love forward. Be well.

Gratitude and Grace

This book exists because of the presence, witness, love, and care of those I am graced to walk beside. Thank you to my beautiful daughter, Cree, who saves my whole heart; my grandsuns Muzari & Yaro, and their dad, Mekell. Thank you to my "day one" loves, Gina T, Jocelyn, Angel, Karma, Nivea, Rachel, Rosesharon, Lucretia, Shelley Nicole, Bob, Amanda, Heidi, and Ambiori. Thank you to the brilliant loves who shared their wisdom and encouraged me during this process: Valerie Boyd, Sonya Renee Taylor, Kerri Kelly, Daniel Coleman, Omisade Burney-Scott, Karen Good Marable, Emanuel Brown, Kate Gerson, and my Rethinc family. Thank you to some of my wonderful teachers: Rev. Dr. Andriette Earl, Joseph Rael, Rasha , JoAnne Dodgson. Thank you to my wonderful agent, Regina Brooks at Serendipity Literary Agency, to my fabulous editors Angela Wix and Sarah Stanton, and to Anastasia Pellouchoud, Jennifer Brown, Tara, Joe Sweeney, Jeff Mack, and all the crew at Sounds True. And thank you, dearest Ash-Lee, for the sound of your voice, for being so deeply beautiful, and for holding me in every way possible.

Glossary

ayahuasca: a medicinal brew made from the bark of a woody vine (*Banisteriopsis caapi* of the family Malpighiaceae) and the leaves of a shrubby plant (*Psychotria viridis* of the family Rubiaceae) of South America, used for centuries by Indigenous peoples from the Amazon (Merriam-Webster and me)

ceremony: a formal act or series of acts prescribed by ritual, protocol, or convention (Merriam-Webster)

divination: the practice of determining the hidden significance or cause of events, sometimes foretelling the future, by various natural, psychological, mystical and other techniques (Encyclopedia Britannica)

Gregorian chant: a simple tune with no regular rhythm that is sung in unison and without accompaniment in services of the Roman Catholic Church (Merriam-Webster)

growing edge: that area of your life where there's still a lot of room for improvement, but you're pushing ahead and stretching the margins of that area every day (street dictionary)

Indigenous: of people inhabiting or existing in a land from the earliest times or from before the arrival of colonists

modality: ways of expressing attitudes, obligations, and intentions; how something exists or happens

multiverse: a collection of potentially diverse, observable universes, each of which would comprise everything that is experimentally accessible by a connected community of observers (Britannica)

perineum: the tiny patch of sensitive skin between your genitals (vaginal opening or scrotum) and anus; it's also the bottom region of your pelvic cavity (Cleveland Clinic)

practice: to do or perform often, customarily, or habitually (Merriam-Webster)

ritual: a formal ceremony or series of acts that is always performed in the same way (Britannica)

sacrum: the part of the spinal column that is directly connected with or forms a part of the pelvis; in humans it consists of five fused vertebrae (Merriam-Webster)

Sanskrit: an ancient Indo-Aryan language that is used in the ancient documents that are the Vedas, composed in what is called Vedic Sanskrit; it is the classical language of India and of Hinduism (Merriam-Webster)

shamanism: spiritual phenomenon centered on the shaman, a person who can access various powers through trance or ecstatic spiritual experience. Although shamans' repertoires vary from one culture to the next, they are typically thought to have the ability to heal the sick, to communicate with the otherworld, and often to escort the souls of the dead to the otherworld (Britannica)

solfeggio frequencies: frequencies that are part of the olden nine-tone scale, believed to have incorporated sacred music (Nature Healing Society)

soul: the spiritual principle embodied in human beings, all rational and spiritual beings, or the universe; the immaterial essence, animating principle, or actuating cause of an individual life (Merriam-Webster)

spirit: an animating or vital principle that gives life to physical organisms (Merriam-Webster)

tribal: of, relating to, or characteristic of a tribe (Merriam-Webster)

visioning: to envision or picture mentally with the mind's eye; an experience in which a personage, thing, or event appears vividly or credibly to the mind, although not actually present (Dictionary.com)

Recommended Resources

This resource section provides information on practitioners and organizations that focus on healing and well-being as well as some treasured books that expand the mind, engage the heart, and lift the spirit.

Resource Guide by Region

National

Abortion Defense Network

Communities served: anyone who needs abortion access
Offerings: legal assistance; a legal helpline
Topics covered: sexual and reproductive justice and gender justice
Website: abortiondefensenetwork.org

Accountability Mapping

Communities served: queer and trans Black, Indigenous, people of color
Offerings: online somatics course on centered accountability
Topics covered: healing justice, transformative justice, gender justice
Website: accountabilitymapping.thinkific.com

Acorn Center for Freedom

Communities served: queer and trans Black, Indigenous, people of color
Offerings: healing arts and spiritual justice practices

Topics covered: healing justice, spirit justice, racial justice, land justice
Website: acorncenter4freedom.com

API Chaya

Communities served: survivors of sexual violence, human trafficking, and domestic violence from Pacific Islander, Native Hawaiian, Asian, and South Asian communities, as well as queer and trans Black, Indigenous, people of color, and immigrant communities
Offerings: culturally specific survivor support services, leadership and skill-building programs, a helpline, community organizing, support groups, creative arts healing
Topics covered: gender justice, healing justice, transformative justice
Website: apichaya.org

Black Feminist Future

Communities served: Black women, girls, and gender expansive people
Offerings: leadership development, movement building, advocacy, resources, organizing programs and schools
Topics covered: gender justice, healing justice, transformative justice
Website: blackfeministfuture.org

Black LGBTQIA+ Migrant Project

Communities served: Black LGBTQIA+
Offerings: national organizing, research, deportation defense, direct support
Regional networks: Oakland, California; New York City; the South; the Upper Midwest (Twin Cities, Chicago, Detroit); Washington DC/DMV
Topics covered: gender justice, racial justice
Website: transgenderlawcenter.org/programs/blmp

The Brown BOI Project

Communities served: masculine of center womyn, women, girls, queer and trans people of people of color
Offerings: trainings, leadership development, financial wellness program, community
Topics covered: economic justice, racial justice, gender justice
Website: brownboiproject.org

Climate Justice Alliance

Communities served: communities that share legacies of racial and economic oppression and social justice organizing
Offerings: network of grassroot movements and organization building local alternatives that center traditional ecological and cultural knowledge
Topics covered: just transition, climate justice
Website: climatejusticealliance.org

COCOA

Communities served: BIPOC
Offerings: language, advocacy, and consulting services within the United States
Topics covered: language justice, disability justice, racial justice
Website: cocoallc.org

Creative Interventions

Communities served: resources for everyday people to end violence
Offerings: tools and resources to help anyone create community-based, collective responses to domestic, family, and sexual violence
Topics covered: gender justice, transformative justice
Website: creative-interventions.org

Familia LGBTQ

Communities served: LGBTQ immigrants
Offerings: leadership development, community building, direct support to migrants, advocacy
Topics covered: racial justice, gender justice
Website: familiatqlm.org

HEAL Food Alliance

Communities served: rural and urban farmers, fishers, farm and food chain workers, Indigenous groups, scientists, public health advocates, policy experts, community organizers, and activists
Offerings: leadership development, community building, resources, skills and knowledge sharing, advocacy, policy change
Topics covered: environmental justice, food justice, health justice
Website: healfoodalliance.org

Health Justice Commons

Communities served: people with disabilities, QTBIPOC
Offerings: health justice training and consultation, healing justice movement building, advocacy, mutual aid, community
Topics covered: racial justice, economic justice, gender justice, disability justice, environmental justice
Website: healthjusticecommons.org

HEARD

Communities served: deaf and hard of hearing community; persons with disabilities
Offerings: grassroots advocacy, community organizing, peer support, mutual aid, education, research
Topics covered: disability justice, abolition, language justice
Website: behearddc.org

Incite!

Communities served: network of radical feminists of color
Offerings: advocacy, educational resources, community
Topics covered: abolition, gender justice, transformative justice
Website: incite-national.org

Language Justice Groups Directory— Collectivizing Language Justice

Offerings: interpretation, translation, trainings, consultation, courses, equipment rental, capacity building, transcription, subtitling, language learning
Topics Covered: language justice, social justice
URL: docs.google.com/spreadsheets/d/1nsqNAgV2qnCfb MYBALXCslDSK7T7JD9kF6x4DBkf0Jw/edit#gid=0

me too.

Communities served: survivors of sexual violence
Offerings: advocacy, community, educational and healing support libraries, leadership training, healing circles, fellowship
Topics covered: healing justice, gender justice
Website: metoomvmt.org

Move to End Violence

Communities served: BIPOC and queer and trans leaders in the antiviolence movement
Offerings: educational resources, community
Topics covered: gender justice, racial justice, healing justice, language justice, disability justice, transformative justice
Website: movetoendviolence.org

Movement Generation

Offerings: political education, movement building, cultural strategy, educational resources
Topics covered: ecological justice, economic justice, disability justice, social justice, just transition and recovery, resilience-based organizing, translocal organizing
Website: movementgeneration.org

National Black Doulas Association

Communities served: BIPOC birthing families
Offerings: trainings, national directory
Topics covered: sexual and reproductive justice, gender justice, racial justice, healing justice
Website: blackdoulas.org

National Latina Institute of Reproductive Justice

Communities served: Latinas and Latinxs
Offerings: advocacy, education, community, movement base-building, leadership development, resources
Regional presence: Florida, New York, Texas, Virginia, Washington, DC
Topics covered: sexual and reproductive justice, rights and health; gender justice; racial justice
Website: latinainstitute.org

National Network of Abortion Funds

Communities served: anyone who needs access to a safe abortion
Offerings: financial support, transportation, childcare, translation, doula services, travel and housing, educational materials, directory
Topics covered: racial justice, economic justice, reproductive justice
Website: abortionfunds.org

National Queer & Trans Therapists of Color Network

Communities served: QTBIPOC
Offerings: educational materials, therapist directory, resource library, mental health funding
Topics covered: healing justice, racial justice, mental health support
Website: nqttcn.com/en/

NDN Collective

Communities served: Indigenous peoples from Turtle Island
Offerings: advocacy, grants, fellowships, community
Topics covered: environmental justice, climate justice, Indigenous people's rights, land justice
Website: ndncollective.org

RAINN (Rape, Abuse & Incest National Network)

Communities served: survivors of sexual violence
Offerings: sexual assault hotline, victim services, public policy, consulting and training, educational materials, research
Website: rainn.org

Raliance

Communities served: network focused on sexual violence prevention
Offerings: training, consulting, advocacy materials, resources for survivors, research, database
Topics covered: sexual and domestic violence
Website: raliance.org

ROOT (Reclaiming Our Own Transcendence)

Communities served: QTBIPOC interpersonal, survivors of sexual violence and harm doers
Offerings: collective repair support, tailored collective healing workshops, resources, educational materials,

People's Healing Conference and Clinic
Topics covered: healing justice, transformative justice, abolition
Website: wetakeroot.com

Transgender Law Center (TLC)
Communities served: transgender and gender non-conforming people, cross-disability justice communities, most specifically Deaf and chronically ill communities
Offerings: legal clinics, help desk and resources, legal strategic litigation, policy advocacy, educational efforts, movement building, program creation for the community
Topics covered: disability justice, gender justice
Website: transgenderlawcenter.org

Translash
Communities served: people who are transgender and gender non-conforming
Offerings: cross-platform media and digital community for trans-affirming content, resources, events
Topics covered: gender justice, social justice, racial justice
Website: translash.org

The Wind & The Warrior
Communities served: healing arts collaborative rooted in liberatory, mindfulness, and Indigenous ancestral wisdom traditions
Website: windandwarrior.com

Women's Earth Alliance
Communities served: grassroots women leaders working for climate and environmental justice
Offerings: training, funding, networks of support
Topics covered: climate justice, gender justice
Website: womensearthalliance.org

California

CIELO's Center for Indigenous Language and Power (CILP)

Location: Los Angeles, California
Communities served: Indigenous migrant communities
Offerings: culture programming, financial solidarity, interpretation services, interpreter training, cultural awareness training
Topics covered: racial justice, language justice
Website: mycielo.org/cilp/

Earthlodge Center for Transformation

Location: Long Beach, California
Communities served: all queer identity peoples, womyn, elders, children and men who recognize and respect the rise of feminine energy on the planet
Offerings: healing resources, earth medicine, and ceremonies
Topics covered: healing justice
Website: earthlodgecenter.org

El/La Para Trans Latinas

Location: San Francisco, California
Communities served: trans Latinas
Offerings: community events, leadership development, advocacy, HIV prevention, PrEP navigation, violence prevention, resource library
Topics covered: gender justice, racial justice
Website: ellaparatranslatinas.org

Indigenous Circle of Wellness

Location: Commerce, California
Communities served: BIPOC
Offerings: sliding scale individual, couple and family counseling that is culturally inclusive and centered in

Indigenous core values
Topics covered: healing justice, racial justice
Website: icowellness.com

Indigenous Regeneration

Location: San Diego, California
Communities served: Indigenous communities in San Diego
Offerings: programming on traditional and contemporary food cultivation; environmental awareness and stewardship; traditional plant education and integration; Indigenous primitive survival skills; healthy expression through music, art and culture; regenerative agriculture concepts; sustainable building techniques
Topics covered: economic justice, environmental justice, land justice, healing justice, Indigenous peoples rights
Website: indigenousregeneration.org

Mirror Memoirs

Location: Los Angeles, California
Communities served: QTBIPOC survivors of child sexual abuse
Offerings: mutual aid fund, community, advocacy, member support, leadership development
Topics covered: abolition, gender justice, transformative justice, disability justice, healing justice
Website: linktr.ee/mirror.memoirs

Restoring Justice for Indigenous Peoples

Location: Sacramento, California
Communities served: survivors of physical and sexual violence, trafficking, former and current sex workers, formerly incarcerated peoples, Indigenous spiritual advisors and leaders, youth, two-spirit relatives, and non-binary individuals in California's rural and urban Indigenous communities

Offerings: direct care and support, advocacy, leadership training
Topics covered: abolition, sexual and reproductive justice, racial justice, Indigenous rights, land justice, healing justice
Website: indigenousjustice.org

Roots of Labor Birth Collective

Location: San Francisco, California
Communities served: all birthing peoples; centering on low-income, BIPOC communities, people with disabilities, incarcerated people, immigrants (regardless of status)
Offerings: educational resources, trainings, skillshares, BIPOC doula circles, doula directory, community
Topics covered: sexual and reproductive justice, racial justice
Website: rootsoflaborbc.com

Translatin@ Coalition

Location: Los Angeles, California
Communities served: transgender, intersex, and gender-nonconforming Latin@ immigrants
Offerings: outreach, case management and referrals, advocacy, leadership development, economic and workforce development, reentry, transition house, legal services, drop-in services, biomedical access, violence prevention
Topics covered: gender justice
Website: translatinacoalition.org/services-in-los-angeles

Northwest

Creative Justice

Location: Seattle, Washington
Communities served: youth most impacted by the school-to-prison-(to-deportation) pipeline

Offerings: relief funding, mentor artist intensive program, leadership gatherings and projects, education and fundraising campaigns
Topics covered: racial justice, abolition, healing justice
Website: creativejusticenw.org

Northeast

Alliance of Black Doulas for Black Mamas

Location: Orange, Durham, Wake, Chatham, and Granville counties in North Carolina
Communities served: Black families
Offerings: doula training program, doula services
Topics covered: sexual and reproductive justice, gender justice, racial justice
Website: leadoula.org

Black Doula Project

Location: Washington, DC, and Baltimore
Communities served: Black families in the District of Columbia and Baltimore City
Offerings: funding to cover birth and postpartum doula services
Topics covered: gender justice, racial justice, reproductive justice and care
Website: blackdoulaproject.com

Haitian Women for Haitian Refugees

Location: Brooklyn, New York
Communities served: Haitian and other Black refugees
Offerings: resilience funds, education, community organizing, leadership development and collective action, crisis intervention, disaster relief, legal clinics

Topics covered: climate justice, racial justice, gender justice, reproductive justice, health justice, social justice, economic justice
Website: haitianrefugees.org

Philadelphia Language Justice Collective

Location: Philadelphia, Pennsylvania
Offerings: interpreter practice, trainings, and interpretation equipment rental
Topics covered: language justice
Website: phillylanguagejusticecollective.wordpress.com

Soul Fire Farm

Location: Petersburg, New York
Communities served: BIPOC
Offerings: food sovereignty programs, fellowship, skillshares, educational resources, trainings
Topics covered: food justice, land justice, racial justice, healing justice, environmental justice
Website: soulfirefarm.org

Tilde Language Services

Location: Lancaster, Pennsylvania
Communities served: BIPOC
Offerings: translation, editing, transcription
Topics covered: language justice
Website: tildelanguage.com/

Southeast

Banchalenguas

Location: New Orleans, Louisiana
Offerings: in-person and virtual interpretation, translation, consulting, and language justice training
Topics covered: language justice
Website: banchalenguas.com

Birthmark Doulas

Location: New Orleans, Louisiana
Communities served: pregnant and parenting people and their families in New Orleans
Offerings: doula services, childbirth education, perinatal health advocacy, lactation services, postpartum doulas, support groups
Topics covered: reproductive justice and care
Website: birthmarkdoulas.com

Center for Participatory Change

Location: Western North Carolina
Communities served: communities most affected by structural inequities, especially Latinx and Black communities
Offerings: popular education, racial equity, language justice
Topics covered: healing justice, language justice, racial justice
Website: cpcwnc.org

Highlander Research and Education Center

Location: New Market, Tennessee
Communities served: people directly impacted in the region
Offerings: movement building, education for action, fiscal sponsorship, fund
Website: highlandercenter.org

Spirit House

Location: Durham, North Carolina
Communities served: Black communities
Offerings: transformative justice training, advocacy, movement building, healing offerings, educational resources

Topics covered: healing justice, racial justice, social justice, transformative justice
Website: spirithouse-nc.org

Transgender Advocates Knowledgeable Empowering (TAKE)

Location: Birmingham, Alabama
Communities served: trans people of color
Offerings: preventive health care, crisis assistance, fund drop-in center, life coaching, street outreach and reentry, legal services, trans-masculine support, homeless shelter, community, freedom school
Topics covered: trans-related issues
Website: takebhm.org

Love Me Unlimited 4 Life

Location: Mississippi
Communities served: transgender community in Mississippi
Offerings: education, advocacy, support
Topics covered: gender justice
Website: unlimitedloveme4life.com

Midwest

Chicago Birthworks Collective

Location: Chicago, Illinois
Communities served: BIPOC birthing people and their families
Offerings: full-circle doula care, classes
Topics covered: gender justice, racial justice, reproductive justice and care
Website: chicagobirthworks.com

Freedom, Inc.

Location: Chicago, Illinois
Communities served: low-income and no-income communities of color
Offerings: direct services, leadership development, community organizing
Topics covered: gender justice, queer justice, Black and Southeast Asian liberation
Website: freedom-inc.org/index.php

Transforming Generations

Location: Saint Paul, Minnesota
Communities served: Hmong and Southeast Asian victims/survivors of gender-based violence
Offerings: advocacy, community awareness, health and wellness, training and education, queer justice program, youth programs, community
Topics covered: gender justice, healing justice, transformative justice
Website: transforminggenerations.org

Southwest

Comal Language Justice Collective

Location: North Texas
Offerings: interpretation, translation, capacity building
Topics covered: language justice
Website: instagram.com/comal.ljc/?hl=en%22

Community Language Cooperative

Location: Englewood, Colorado
Offerings: interpretation, translation, language justice training, consultation
Topics covered: language justice
Website: communitylanguagecoop.com/

Organización Latina Trans in Texas

Location: Houston, Texas
Communities served: trans Latinx community
Offerings: temporary housing, community organizing, legal services, gender-affirming care, health services, trans and queer celebrations
Topics covered: gender justice, healing justice, transformative justice
Website: latinatranstexas.org

Southern Movement Assembly

Location: the South
Communities served: multiracial, multi-issue, multigenerational movement alliance of grassroots organizations across the South
Offerings: movement building, network, advocacy
Topics covered: social justice
Website: southtosouth.org

Books I Love

Dear family, this is an ever-expanding list as I am always discovering new works by amazing people. This list encompasses the books I have been reading for the last few years. I am so grateful for this medicine. Please send an email through ginabreedlove.com to share books that you have been reading that support your well-being. We will read those books too and share them on our website.

Anzaldua, Gloria. *Light in the Dark/Luz en lo Oscuro: Rewriting Identity, Spirituality, Reality. Durham,* North Carolina: Duke University Press Books, 2015.

Beyer, Tamiko, Destiny Hemphiill, and Lisbeth White, eds. *Poetry as Spellcasting: Poems, Essays, and Prompts for Manifesting Liberation and Reclaiming Power.* Berkeley, California: North Atlantic Books, 2023.

Bourgeault, Cynthia. *The Wisdom Jesus: Transforming Heart and Mind—A New Perspective on Christ and His Message.* Boston, Massachusetts: Shambhala, 2008.

Boyd, Valerie, ed. *Bigger Than Bravery: Black Resilience and Reclamation in a Time of Pandemic.* Wilmington, North Carolina: Lookout Books, 2022.

brown, adrienne maree. *Emergent Strategy: Shaping Change, Changing Worlds.* Chico, California: AK Press, 2017.

Burney-Scott, Omisade. *Messages From The Menopausal Multiverse.* Black Girl's Guide to Surviving Menopause, 2021.

Cameron, Anne. *Daughters of Copper Woman.* British Columbia, Canada: Harbour Publishing, 2002.

Carruthers, Charlene A. *Unapologetic: A Black, Queer, and Feminist Mandate for Radical Movements.* Boston, Massachusetts: Beacon Press, 2019.

Chen, Ching-In, Jai Dulani, and Leah Lakshmi Piepzna-Samarasinha, eds. *The Revolution Starts at Home: Confronting Intimate Violence Within Activist Communities.* Chico, California: AK Press, 2016.

Crass, Chris. *Towards Collective Liberation: Anti-Racist Organizing, Feminist Praxis, and Movement Building Strategy.* Binghamton, New York: PM Press, 2013.

Creative Interventions Toolkit: A Practical Guide to Stop Interpersonal Violence. Chico, California: AK Press, 2021.

Dennis, Monica and Priscilla Hung, eds. *Infinite Rotations: Reflections from the Move to End Violence Community 2010–2022.* Move to End Violence, 2023.

Dixon, Ejeris and Leah Lakshmi Piepzna-Samarasinha, eds. *Beyond Survival: Strategies and Stories from the Transformative Justice Movement.* Chico, California: AK Press, 2020.

Emoto, Masaru. *The Hidden Messages in Water.* New York: Atria Books, 2005.

Garza, Alicia. *The Purpose of Power, How We Come Together When We Fall Apart.* One World/Random House, 2021.

Gumbs, Alexis Pauline. *Undrowned: Black Feminist Lessons from Marine Mammals (Emergent Strategy, 2).* Chico, California: AK Press, 2020.

Hersey, Tricia. *Rest Is Resistance: A Manifesto.* New York: Little, Brown Spark, 2022.

hooks, bell. *all about love: New Visions*. New York: William Morrow
Paperbacks, 2018.

Kaba, Mariame. *We Do This 'Til We Free Us: Abolitionist Organizing
and Transforming Justice.* Chicago, Illinois: Haymarket Books, 2021.

Kaba, Mariame and Shira Hassan. *Fumbling Towards Repair: A
Workbook for Community Accountability Facilitators.* Chicago,
Illinois: Project NIA, 2019.

Kelley, Robin D. G. *Freedom Dreams: The Black Radical Imagination.*
Boston, Massachusetts: Beacon Press, 2022.

Kelly, Kerri. *American Detox: The Myth of Wellness and How We Can
Truly Heal. Berkeley, California:* North Atlantic Books, 2022.

Kimmerer, Robin Wall. *Braiding Sweetgrass: Indigenous Wisdom,
Scientific Knowledge and the Teachings of Plants.* Minneapolis,
Minnesota: Milkweed Editions, 2015.

Lipsky, Laura van Dernoot and Connie Burk. *Trauma Stewardship:
An Everyday Guide to Caring for Self While Caring for Others.*
Oakland, California: Berrett-Koehler Publishers, 2009.

Macy, Joanna. *World as Lover, World as Self: Courage for Global Justice
and Ecological Renewal.* Berkeley, California: Parallax Press, 2007.

Mason-John, Valerie. *Detox Your Heart: Meditations for Healing
Emotional Trauma.* Somerville, Massachusetts: Wisdom
Publications, 2017.

Mitchell, Sherri. *Sacred Instructions: Indigenous Wisdom for Living Spirit-
Based Change.* Berkeley, California: North Atlantic Books, 2018.

Morales, Aurora Levins. *Remedios: Stories of Earth and Iron from the History
of Puertorriqueñas.* Boston, Massachusetts: Beacon Press, 1998.

O'Donohue, John. *To Bless the Space Between Us: A Book of Blessings.*
New York: Doubleday, 2008.

Owens, Lama Rod. *Love and Rage: The Path of Liberation through
Anger.* Berkeley, California: North Atlantic Books, 2020.

Page, Cara and Erica Woodland. *Healing Justice Lineages: Dreaming
at the Crossroads of Liberation, Collective Care, and Safety.* Berkeley,
California: North Atlantic Books, 2023.

Penniman, Leah. *Farming While Black: Soul Fire Farm's Practical Guide to Liberation on the Land.* Chelsea, Vermont: Chelsea Green Publishing, 2018.

Rael, Joseph. *being & vibration: Entering the New World.* Millichap Books, 2022.

Rasha. Oneness. Tamil Nadu, India: Earthstar Press, 2006.

Schaefer, Carol. *Grandmothers Counsel the World: Women Elders Offer Their Vision for Our Planet.* Boston, Massachusetts: Trumpeter, 2006.

Simmons, Aishah Shahidah, ed. *Love WITH Accountability: Digging up the Roots of Child Sexual Abuse.* Chico, California: AK Press, 2019.

Taylor, Sonya Renee. *The Body Is Not an Apology: The Power of Radical Self-Love.* Oakland, California: Berrett-Koehler Publishers, 2018.

Tyson, Neil deGrasee. *Astrophysics for People in a Hurry.* New York: W. W. Norton & Company, 2017.

VanDyke, Lucretia. *African American Herbalism: A Practical Guide to Healing Plants and Folk Traditions.* New York: Ulysses Press, 2022.

Vega, Marta Moreno. *The Altar of My Soul: The Living Traditions of Santeria.* New York: One World, 2001.

Walker, Alice. *Gathering Blossoms Under Fire: The Journals of Alice Walker, 1965–2000.* New York: Simon & Schuster, 2022.

Williams, Rev. angel Kyodo, Lama Rod Owens, and Jasmine Syedullah, PhD. *Radical Dharma: Talking Race, Love, and Liberation.* Berkeley, California: North Atlantic Books, 2016.

Williams, Justine M. and Eric Holt- Giménez, eds. *Land Justice: Re-imagining Land, Food, and the Commons in the United States.* Pasadena, California: Food First Books, 2017.

Wong, Alice. *Disability Visibility: First-Person Stories from the Twenty-First Century.* New York: Vintage, 2020.

About the Author

gina Breedlove (she/they/Grace) is from the people's republic of Brooklyn. She tours the world sharing the Vibration of Grace™ as a vocalist, composer, actor, playwright, sound healer, and grief doula. gina began her walk with music and spirit at age nine, singing in her family's church in Apalachicola, Florida. When she was sixteen, she sang background for the incomparable Phyllis Hyman; toured with legendary artist and activist Harry Belafonte; worked on two Spike Lee joints; released two records, *Open Heart* and *Language of Light*; and is an original cast member of the Broadway production of *The Lion King*. gina has been sharing the medicine of sound and the power of grief-letting for over twenty years, working with people and organizations around the world. She is grateful for this life of service, practice, fellowship, and love. You can learn more about gina's work at ginabreedlove.com.

About Sounds True

Sounds True was founded in 1985 by Tami Simon with a clear mission: to disseminate spiritual wisdom. Since starting out as a project with one woman and her tape recorder, we have grown into a multimedia publishing company with a catalog of more than 3,000 titles by some of the leading teachers and visionaries of our time, and an ever-expanding family of beloved customers from across the world.

In more than three decades of evolution, Sounds True has maintained its focus on our overriding purpose and mission: to wake up the world. We offer books, audio programs, online learning experiences, and in-person events to support your personal growth and awakening, and to unlock our greatest human capacities to love and serve.

At SoundsTrue.com you'll find a wealth of resources to enrich your journey, including our weekly *Insights at the Edge* podcast, free downloads, and information about our nonprofit Sounds True Foundation, where we strive to remove financial barriers to the materials we publish through scholarships and donations worldwide.

To learn more, please visit SoundsTrue.com/freegifts or call us toll-free at 800.333.9185.

Together, we can wake up the world.

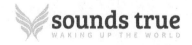

sounds true
WAKING UP THE WORLD